Bioenergy Economy

Bioenergy Economy

A Methodological Study on Bioenergy-Based Therapies

Farzad Goli, MD

With a foreword by
Prof. Micheal Wirsching
and
Prof. Carl Eduard Scheidt

To order additional copies of this book, contact:
Xlibris Corporation
1-888-795-4274
www.Xlibris.com
Orders@Xlibris.com
82012

Foreword

Over the last decades, methods of complementary medicines have become an integral part of the health services in many medical centers. This development reflects the growing awareness of the shortcomings of the biomedicine paradigm, which is based primarily on the biosciences. Within Western medicine, a shift toward the broadening of the perspective to include also the complex interaction of biological and psychosocial factors in the understanding of health and disease was put forward by psychosomatic medicine. According to this view, a patient-centered approach should be a core issue of medicine. The biopsychosocial model as suggested by Engel is the theoretical framework, which helped to organize the growing knowledge about the interrelationship between biological and psychosocial interactions in the development of illnesses and their treatments. Complementary medicine was an important ally of psychosomatic medicine from its beginning. The common ground between complementary medicine and psychosomatic medicine is the patient-centered approach instead of the disease-oriented approach. Both complementary medicine and psychosomatics both are focusing on salutogenesis—the maintenance and development of resources instead of pathology and pathogenesis. There is also a substantial overlap of treatment methods. Yoga and the other bioenergy-based healing systems, such as Reiki and Qigong, are methods to increase self-awareness and self-knowledge, and they are in wide use in psychosomatic treatment. However, despite the widespread clinical use of these methods, a conceptual framework, which illuminates the common roots of these approaches, their sociocultural background, their theoretical and conceptual implications, and also their differences, is still a desideratam. It is the merit of Dr. Goli's book to address this issue in a thorough and profound way.

One reason that makes the illumination of the basic concepts of complementary medicine a challenge is the fact that there is a great variety of different methods, which have to be integrated and which have considerable differences with regard to their theoretical and their sociocultural background. Their cultural origin stems from Western philosophy and science as well as from Eastern religious and philosophical concepts and healing traditions. The theoretical challenge to strive for a unifying framework for such various and diverging concepts and ideas makes *bioenergy economy* a unique and extremely stimulating reading.

Perhaps complementary medicine, by opening up its theoretical concepts to different cultural systems, can contribute to a new paradigm of medicine: a paradigm, which is integrating the healing experiences and the theoretical concepts of treatment in various cultures. Perhaps it is not accidental that such an integration is developing in Iran—a cultural context, which for long, has played the role of a bridge between the Eastern and Western cultural discourses.

The concept of "energy," which in the work of Dr. Goli plays an essential role as a basic concept for understanding and integrating the view on physiological and psychological processes, has also played an important role in Western theories. Freud made an extensive use of this concept in the metapsychology of psychoanalysis and also considered the metaphor of psychic energy as a concept for bridging the gap between the biological matrix and psychological processes. In his book, Dr. Goli exemplifies the richness of this concept from various perspectives, using scientific theories as well as drawing from religious and mythological concepts. However, the reader is also provided with relevant data on the empirical evidence supporting the fact that methods of complementary medicines are well-compatible with evidence-based medicine in that their effectiveness can be tested in comparable ways as other treatment methods.

At the beginning of a three-year perspective of cooperation on teaching training and research between the universities of Freiburg and the International University of Medical Sciences in Esfahan, which is supported by a grant of the German Government (DAAD), we consider Dr. Golis's contribution as an excellent basis to develop a truly intercultural dialogue and discussion. The book demands and supports on the side of its readers a capacity for integration. It provides us with a text that has multiple layers stemming from different cultural contexts, is rich and complex, and at the same time is not lacking in clarity. Complementary medicine and especially energy-based therapies are clearly an intercultural endeavor, and this might turn out to be their greatest strength.

Prof. Dr. Michael Wirsching
Psychosomatic Department
Albert Ludwig University Freiburg

Prof. Dr. Carl E. Scheidt
Psychosomatic Department
Albert Ludwig University Freiburg
and Thure von Uexküll Hospital

A Word to the Reader

After twenty years of Ulysses-like wandering and experiencing different healing methods, from oriental tradition to Sufism, alchemy, and symbology and also learning and teaching psychosomatic medicine techniques such as hypnotherapy, relaxation therapy and meditation and the clinical experience of thousands of patients with chronic physical and psychological problems or the ones-only-visited-for-consciousness evaluation, I discerned a common pattern underlying all these methodological and morphological variations, and a conceptual matrix was formed in my mind. I cannot by any means claim that this is a punctilious and overarching pattern, like satellite maps, and it is more like an ancient analogical map depicted on papyrus or hide with its knots and slots. This book seeks to present an unitarian biofield model in its primary version.

An ever-rising turn to complementary and alternative medicine has been developed in the recent two decades. Several survey studies have demonstrated that 45 to 80 percent of population both in developing and developed countries use these services. Energy medicine has had a considerable contribution in this domain of health services. Several reports of World Health Organization and national institutes of health show the importance of these two overlapping and related groups of complementary therapies.

Notwithstanding the reports and studies on cost-effectiveness of energy-based therapies, increasing demand of these services and active role of clients in these healing systems, there is no clinical and methodological model to integrate several healing techniques into one consistent health system. These demands persuaded my colleagues and me to establish bioenergy economy as an integrative health model.

A large variety of energy-based therapies exists; extend from traditional methods as Qigong and Reiki to modern techniques such as therapeutic touch and polarity therapy, from psychosomatic methods, such as yoga and tai chi, to biophysical methods like acupuncture and homeopathy, and from the local-mechanical techniques, such as artificial energy healing, to the nonlocal parapsychological techniques, such as prayer and distant healing.

Although this model provides a methodological framework for expounding and applying all of the energy-based therapies, bioenergy economy, however, focuses on autogenic and communicative techniques and grounds an integral clinical program in this field. As such, bioenergy economy can be recognized as a psychosomatic approach to energy medicine which manages bioenergy in intra/inter/transpersonal domains toward higher health and consciousness evolution.

This unitarian health model is named "economy" instead of "therapy" because of three main reasons: first is to avoid medicalization trends upon which "therapy" is based. The second one is related to reductionistic inductions of "therapy doctor in" which reduce life, communication, and healing to function, clinical reasoning, and treatment, and the last one concerns etymology of the term of "economy" which means management of *Oikos* or home. The bio/psycho/social systems are our home, and bioenergy in each form (material, energetic, or informational) should be organized toward self-actualization and a full-function life. On the other hand, bioenergy economy is related to the Freudian term of "libidinal economy" and economy of the "organic energy" in Wilhelm Reich's body psychoanalysis. Thus, although this model is predicated on the most recent scientific and clinical findings in this field, it does not present a reductionistic view. Bioenergy economy explains healing systems as communicative and systematic techniques which coordinate mind and body, man and nature, and medicine and life.

It should be noted that healing traditions, which were always nonanalytical and qualitative methods, originate from various cultures and religions. So to enjoy their experiences without making the life of our customers more complicated and conflict and linking these cost-effective services to integrative health system, we have to adopt two essential strategies:

1- Distinguish the effective elements from cultural and ideological ones.
2- Defining the mechanisms and clinical applications on the basis of a single methodological pattern.

I am not sure to what extent I have been successful in this regard, but as you will, I have tried to follow these two rules in defining the fundamental physical and physiological mechanisms of bioenergy-based therapies, as well as introducing bioenergetic integrative health model.

In this model, human condition is depicted as a stream of transformation and interaction of consciousness-information-energy-matter in the intra/inter/transpersonal communications, and health and illness are defined as meaningfulness or meaninglessness of these biosemiotic events. Each disease, from this viewpoint, could be explained simply as a specific disturbance in energy-information flow. It may be embodied in the form of organic dysfunctions and deformities, and as such, it can alter the state of consciousness. Healing, in this model, is an intentional energy-information flow which harmonizes the organism and reorganizes the biosemiosis flow.

Any of the known methods of bioenergy healing can fulfill this intervention from a specific point of view, and if employed on a common clinical and physiological basis, they can yield synergetic effects. In this book, I have primarily introduced bioenergy economy as a methodological basis for bioenergy-based therapies, and I hope I can deliberate more punctiliously on its applied aspects in my next book.

Systemic approaches to health and life, such as biopsychosocial model of George Engel and biosemiotical psychosomatic theory of Thure Von Uexkuell, are the other theoretical premises of bioenergy economy. Such a systemic approach is different from biomedical approach of energy medicine. Energy medicine explores bioenergetic phenomena only on the base of physics; biochemistry and physiology biopsychosocial resourses and their effects are reduced to electromagnetic actions and events. The analytic approach of energy medicine is indispensable to explain bioenergetic phenomena, but we require a synthetic approach to clarify systemic initiators and consequences.

Bioenergy economy is a biopsychosocial paradigm of energy medicine which studies bioenergetic phenomena in the biopsychosociospritual matrix, quantitatively and qualitatively. These two complementary approach are considered under tow new technical term, *Qikinetics* and *Qidynamics*.

Qikinetics concentrates on quantitative analysis *(in vitro/in vivo)* of direct effects of bioenergetic factors on the functions of living systems, but Qidynamics deals with biopsychosocial context which generates and conducts bioenergetic pluses and so determines responses to them.

While energy medicine concentrates on Qikinetics, bioenergy economy seeks to posit a theoretical framework for working out both Qikinetical and Qidynamical aspects of biofield emissions and receptions.

This work owes to numerous scientists and researchers. Unfortunately, I could not fit them in the conceptual network of this book. However, I specially thank Dr. James Oschman, whose comprehensive and inspiring studies illuminated my path since ten years.

I would also like to thank my kind wife, Dr. Mahboubeh Farzanegan, my dear friends Reza Abdollahi and Reza Jouharifard for collecting the experiences of practitioners and the data and drafts and also Dr. Alireza Rezaei and Dr. Alireza Gholamrezaei for translation of some parts of the book. I also thank Ms. Azadeh Okhovat, who took the trouble of typesetting and management of the references.

Moreover, I am deeply indebted to Dr. Alireza Fakhrkonandeh, who helped me in time to proofread and edit the text.

I am boundlessly beholden to erudite Prof. Michael Wirsching and Prof. Carl Scheidt for their meticulous reading of the book and their generous and illuminating preface to the book. I also wish to express my appreciation and gratitude to Mrs. Ghazal Karimpour for her unfaltering pursuit of publication procedures.

Considering my limited knowledge and experience and also novelty of this field of knowledge, I am sure that there are many deficiencies and drawbacks in this work. I hope your valuable feedback can help me to improve the next editions of this book.

Farzad Goli
Isfahan, 2010

Contents

Keywords: Mind-Body Medicine, Complementary and Alternative Medicine, Energy Medicine, Energy-Based Therapies, Transpersonal Psychology

Chapter *I*

Theoretical and Philosophical Bases

During different eras and in several cultures, human beings have used various energy-based methods to maintain and improve health.

Nowadays, in spite of their intuitive, practice-based, and culture-based methods, traditional healing systems have been examined experimentally, and some of their hypotheses have been confirmed.

Whether the focus is on the ancient healing systems, which consider such concepts as Chi, Prana, or Ki, or on the modern science, which considers concepts such as the balance of chemical energy, as in pH balance or serotonin level, healing systems have long place value on the balancing of energy (Rotan & Ospina-Kammerer 2007).

Thus, energy medicine can be employed effectively in health-care coverage as a basic science for explaining medical phenomena in the basic level of organisms and so as a kind of complementary medicine:

There are two methods to discuss the theoretical and philosophical bases of energetic approaches to health. First, to postulate the positions of the founders and practitioners of these methods, this patently, would not be devoid of analogical dispositions and ideological predilections. The other one is to be discussed with modern, valid theoretical models, and trying to understand the real situation of this theoretical and clinical model in modern health discourse with a meta-analytic and critical view.

In this study, we have chosen the second method and tried to understand the relationships between the energetic approaches to health in the biopsychosocial framework, their explanation of human condition, and the horizons that have opened up human health and wealth.

Nurses have been integrating energetic healing modalities in their practice for decades. Although public interest and demand for such healing have grown exponentially, the research available to support the use of these modalities is limited (Mansour et al. 1999). Several literature reviews demonstrate that bioenergetic interventions produce positive results (e.g., Crawford, Leaver & Mahoney 2006; Wardell & Engebretson 2006).

However, study design is beset by the several challenges encountered: Energetic modalities are difficult to validate, proscribe, and measure (Potter 2007).

Developing inclination of health providers and consumers to energy-based healing systems, such as Reiki, healing touch and energy psychology, clinical and paraclinical evidences on cost-effectiveness of these interventions, and several problems in research designing in this domain, convinces us to organize these experiences in an integrative and methodological model.

Regarding these theoretical models, researchers and practitioners of these fields can perform in higher coordination with health service systems and also develop their educational programs more scientifically and effectively.

Energy-Based Healing Systems

Energy medicine is a broad experimental field of knowledge predicated on the belief that "in addition to a system of physical and biochemical processes, the human being is made up of a complex system of energy." Clinically, energy medicine is used every day in conventional medicine to diagnose and treat various conditions with methods such as radiation therapy, ultrasound, electrical muscle stimulation, and pacemakers. In addition to these more familiar techniques, there are a lot of methods whose exact mechanisms have been more difficult to identify with available instruments. They are based on the belief that we are all surrounded by a field of energy that flows through and around us and is in a constant and continuous interaction with the environment. In a state of wellness, energy flows freely. These methods may include diagnosis and healing that are less direct, or at a distance, from the intended subject.

Various healings are described in the Bible and other spiritual works all over the world. The "laying on of hands" (also known as therapeutic touch and healing touch) was practiced by Jesus.

The earliest writing describing the human energy field in Chinese culture dates back to 4,000-5,000 years in the *Yellow Emperor's Canon of Medicine*. The first textbook on internal medicine described the movement of qi in the body along meridians, or energy meridians, and its relationship to health. Electricity from electric eels, used for healing the sick, was first documented about 2750 BC (Little 2004).

The first recorded mention of "vital" energy in Western literature was by the Pythagoreans around 500 BC *Vis medicatrix naturae*, or the healing power of nature, was described in Greece by Hippocrates (460-377 BC), who referred to using his hands to "pull and draw" aches and impurities away from his patients. Paracelsus reported "a healing energy that radiates within and around man like a luminous sphere." He maintained that this energy could cause and cure disease, work from a distance, and be influenced by magnets, planets, and stars. Some of the theories and practices of contemporary energy medicine reflect these earlier beliefs.

Baggott (1999) in *The Encyclopedia of Energy Healing* introduced following energy medicine techniques: acupuncture, acupressure, Qigong, tai chi, aikido, yoga, polarity therapy, therapeutic touch, healing touch, Reiki, homeopathy, color, sound, light therapy, and prayer. Some of these healing systems in their own turn subsume several styles and schools, but in our study we consider only common aspects of these systems. In recent decades, some innovative methods have been presented, especially in energy psychology field such as, thought field therapy (TFT), applied kinesthesiology, and emotional freedom technique (EFT).

These techniques work through the biofield (auras), energy centers (chakras) and energy pathways (meridians). Many of these methods utilize verbal affirmation protocols, and subjective scales, in tandem with tapping methods targeted at meridians or chakras, and they promise rapid somato-emotional release for a wide range of physical and emotional problems, such as addiction disorders, PTSD, and allergies. Empirical evidence of the safety and efficacy of many energy psychology approaches is still being established (Little 2004).

In the ensuing sections, we present brief introductions to the most important bioenergy-based methods:

- **Homeopathy**
  The homeopathy method was developed and elaborated by Samuel Hahnemann, MD (1755-1843), a German physician, chemist, and well-known author. He coined the term *homeopathy* to describe his method of applying remedies with the power to resonate with the illness as self-healing responses. According to him, epistemological laws of homeopathy are:

  - Let likes be cured by likes.
  - Healing is the consequence of the whole organism.
  - All healing is essentially self-healing.

  And clinical laws of homeopathy are:

  - *Proving*: ascertaining the therapeutic properties of medicinal substances.
  - *The totality of symptoms*: illness is primarily a disturbance of the vital force and manifests itself as a totality of physical, mental, and emotional responses which is unique to each patient.
  - *The single remedy*: one remedy at a time for an individual patient.
  - *The minimum dose*: as homeopathic remedies stimulate an ailing self-healing mechanism rather than redress a specific abnormality, large or prolonged doses are seldom required and even might undermine the effect (Jacobs & Moskowitz 2002).
  - *The ultrahigh dilution remedies of homeopathy* are vibrational medicines which induce a special energetic pattern similar to illness vibrational pattern to provoke fetal force.

  Chemical tests cannot discern homeopathic remedies and only physical tests such as spectroscopy distinguish specific crystal patterns of these vibrational medicines (Endler & Schulte 1994; Jackson & Mantasch 1996).
  Recent clinical trials have suggested a positive treatment association between homeopathic medicines and the treatment of allergic rhinitis,

fibrositis, asthma, rheumatoid arthritis, hypertension, influenza, ileus, stroke, migraine, insomnia, myalgia, etc (Ernst & Resch 1995; Kleijnen, Knipschild & ter 1991).

- **Acupuncture**

Acupuncture is a modality of treatment derived from East Asian Medicine, although originating from China, which involves stimulation of specific body points by insertion and manipulation of fine needles. When practiced in a context informed by East Asian Medicine, acupuncture is often coupled with other techniques and modalities of traditional Chinese medicine.

Acupuncture facilitates innate healing by stimulating the points. Points are chosen based on the patient's symptoms and their association with East Asian Medicine's common patterns of disharmony, as well as empirical knowledge of disease states and their relation with specific meridians, organs, and areas of the body. Palpation along meridians enhances precise location of important known points and patterns of points requiring needling. Research has demonstrated that bioelectrical and biomechanical activity at points treated by acupuncture distinguishes these sites from surrounding tissues. Acupuncture relieves pain by reducing inflammation, promoting healing, and enhancing immune response. Acupuncture aids the body in resolving acute disorders like common cold, flu, or bronchitis, and chronic problems such as musculoskeletal and neurologic problems. Osteoarthritis (Berman et al. 1999; Haslam 2001; Kleijnen, Knipschild & ter 1991), migraine (Allais et al. 2002; Liguori et al. 2000), rehabilitation of stroke (Naeser et al. 1992), myofascial pain (Birch & Jamison 1998; Nielson & Hammerschlag 2004), allergies and asthma (Joos et al. 2000; Shapira et al. 2002), addiction (Avants et al. 2000; Bier et al. 2002), gynecologic problems such as pregnancy nausea (Knight et al. 2001), and pain and duration of labor (Skilnand, Fossen & Heiberg 2002) may improve or convalesce completely with acupuncture treatment.

- **Acupressure**

Acupressure is the application of the fingers to acupuncture points on the body, or "acupuncture without needles." It is predicated on the same bioenergy meridian system and more or less similar clinical indications. Interruptions in the flow of qi occasion functional aberrations associated with the related meridians: These interruptions can be released by the application of needles or fingers.

Repeated stress in turn causes a layering of tension at a point which is termed the *local point* as a frame of reference. Other related tender points are referred to as *distal points*. Deep pressure applied to the point ultimately brings about a release, and the tension dissipates (Coughlin 2002).

Several pressure-point therapies such as reflexology, shiatsu, touch for health, and Tui Na work on a similar basis with different arrangement of techniques (Ina & Chrisman 2001).

Myofascial release in acupressure and other pressure-point massages are sometimes accompanied by emotional releases as painful memories are brought to consciousness (Coughlin 2002).

- **Qigong**

Qigong is translated as "Qi exercise." It is also known as "longevity method" or "breathing exercise." Medical Qigong for health and healing consists primarily of meditation, physical movements, and breathing exercise.

Qigong is a term that has become popular only in the twentieth century, in fact, adverts to a large group of ancient Chinese healing arts that have been called many things over thousands of years. The foundation of these healing arts lies in the cosmic concept and naturalism of Taoism, in which the concepts and philosophy of Confucianism and Buddhism are incorporated. These concepts were further elaborated and substantiate in theory and methods by many ingenious healers, scholars, and physicians throughout the dynasties of China (Loh 1999).

Qigong is not knowledge, a "skill," or a kind of "work." It is a ceaseless practice and quest to affect harmony between mind and body through persistent physical, mental, moral, and spiritual training methods. There are more than 5,000 styles of Qigong counted by the Chinese government, and each has its own history and training method for specific purposes. Some emphasize visualization, others use movements. Not everyone applies "breathing method." The Tienjin Chinese Medicine Academy has suggested applying different styles of Qigong for different medical conditions (Zhang 1993).

Awareness of qi sensations in the body and intentional guide of qi is the essence of this method.

This therapy has a limited number of applications on a large scale, because the number of skilled Qigong masters is limited.

Qigong is one energy healing intervention used to prevent and cure ailments and to improve health through regular practice (National Center for Complementary and Alternative Medicine, Sancier 1996) Qigong can be divided up into two categories: internal and external. Internal Qigong refers to a self-training method without a practitioner to achieve optimal health in both mind and body (Chen & Yeung 2002, Sancier 1996). External Qigong refers to the process by which Qigong practitioners, who have mastered the technique, direct their qi energy to relieve pain or remedy other illnesses (Lee, Pittler & Ernst 2008).

External Qigong resembles other energy healing modalities such as therapeutic touch, Reiki, and healing touch in a number of respects (ibid).

Several studies on medical Qigang confirm its antiaging effects (Kemp 2004; Kuang et al. 1991), as well as positive effects on hypertension (Wang et al.), pain control (Jang et al. 2004; Lee et al. 2003; Lee, Pittler & Ernst 2008; Yang, Kim & Lee 2005), osteoporosis (Xu & Wang), and cancer (Chen & Yeung 2002; Loh 1999; Sun & Zhao).

- **Tai chi**

Certain breathing and movement techniques have been found to affect the flow of energy, or qi, in the body, in specific ways.

Qi is what animates us and what generates life. To put it plainly, it is generated from the air we breathe and the food and liquids we consume—which is known as postnatal qi—and prental qi, which we received from our parents (Adler & Roberts 2006).

The therapeutic benefits of tai chi are likely to emanate from its emphasis on balance and harmony, continuous slow movements, rhythmic flexion of the lower limbs, extension of the upper body, the symmetrical arm motion, and the constant shifting of weight. Tai chi appears to be a useful adjunctive therapy for patients with arthritis (Kirsteins, Dietz &

Hwang 1991), cardiovascular diseases (Channer et al. 1996), and postural instability in the elderly (Tse & Bailey 1992).

- **Yoga**

The discipline of yoga can be said to date back to 4,000 years ago to the Indus valley. It is an essential component of Ayurveda, one of the oldest complete medical systems in the world. Traditionally, regular yoga practice is believed to unite body, mind, and spirit, thereby enhancing health and quality of life (Russell 2002).

Yoga, as an energetic approach to health, enhances and evokes bioenergy in a long-term and complex program including movements/postures/(asana), breathing exercises (Pranayama), mental skills (Dharana, Diana), and enhancement of awareness of energetic changes and centers in the body (Kandalini Yoga) (Krishna 2000; Udupa 1983).

Biopsychosocial interventions in yogic sciences are different techniques for maintaining, promoting, and organizing "Prana" (vital energy). In yoga, life is Prana plus matter; and health and disease are defined by quantity and quality (equilibrium) of intra/inter/transpersonal Prana (Goli 2003b).

Most participants consent that regular yoga practice heightens flexibility (both physical and mental) improves posture and augments strength and balance. Regular practice also provides an enjoyable means of managing stress and offers a sense of personal involvement, even control, in maintaining or improving health. Although poses have been used in association with specific maladies for millennia, yoga therapy has not generally been considered disease-specific. Regular yoga practice can be beneficial to people with a variety of health problems, including: asthma (Birkel & Edgren 2000), headaches, chronic pain (Nespor 1991), hypertension (Murugesan, Govindarajulu & Bera 2000), depression and anxiety (Janakiramaiah et al. 2000; Ray et al. 2001), insomnia, dysmenorrheal, irritable bowel syndrome, fatigue (Greenfield 2002), lower back pain and other musculoskeletal problems (Sherman et al. 2005;Williams et al. 2005), fibromyalgia, osteoarthritis, and carpal tunnel syndrome (Garfinkel & Schumacher Jr. 2000; Garfinkel et al. 1994;1998).

Yoga may not offer participants a cure for their ailments, but its practice can help people create balance in their lives and boost the quality of life.

• Reiki

Reiki was developed in Japan by Dr. Mikao Usui (1865-1926), a theologian minister, president of Doshisha University, Kyoto. He designed this healing system on the basis of ancient Tibetan sutras (holy writings), describing the use of universal life energy for healing through the laying on of hands. Reiki developed basically as a self-healing program which is activated by:

- Attunement: initiation and alignment of life energy field
- Disciple—master relationship
- Fivefold ethical principles (see appendix A)

According to Reiki tradition, the ability to access and transfer energy is predicated on the attunement process. Master, a more organized energy field, works as a pacemaker for disciple, and during their connection entrains his/her energy field and finally can experience a new state of life energy organization which is achieved and established via daily self-healing training and meditation.

There are three levels of Reiki training which are initiated with three attunements. Completion of the first level renders one a first-degree Reiki practitioner, qualified to treat self, family, and friends only. Completion of the second degree qualifies a Reiki practitioner to treat patients. After completing the third degree, a practitioner becomes a Reiki master and is made eligible to teach other practitioners as well as treat patients (Hurwitz 2001).

In classic Reiki, after the first level, each individual can begin self-healing program, but in addition to this active form of Reiki she/he can practice hands-on Reiki for the others. Reiki's interventions are attunement, ethical observance, hands-on/off technique, and distance healing.

Due to simplicity, effectiveness, and active role of Reiki clients, it is exceedingly developing and a large number of non-Reiki techniques have been presented under the name of Reiki.

A typical Reiki session lasts sixty to ninety minutes and treats the entire body. However, there can be treatments of shorter duration or treatments solely focused on specific areas. The patient is usually in a prone position, although the treatment can take place with the patient in a sitting position. To ensure the free flow of energy, the patient does not cross his or her arms or legs, as this may obstruct the energetic flow. The patient wears loose comfortable clothing, with shoes, eyeglasses, and sometimes even belts or jewelry removed.

Similar to therapeutic touch and healing touch, in Reiki the practitioner begins a therapeutic session by centering, with the intention of the patient's highest good. Although a patient's history may be taken, Reiki differs from therapeutic touch and healing touch in that in Reiki, often no initial physical or energetic assessment is made. Once the patient is in a comfortable position, the Reiki practitioner uses Japanese symbols (kanji) and a sequence of hand positions to transfer energy to the patient. With fingers gently held together and palms down, the practitioner's hands are placed lightly on the patient, beginning with the head and then moving down the body. During these hand placements, universal life energy is said to flow through the practitioner and transfer from the practitioner's hands to the patient, to balance the patient's energy where needed. Each hand position is held for approximately five minutes, or longer, if the practitioner senses continued need of flow. Unlike therapeutic touch and healing touch, Reiki is traditionally practiced "hands-on," although "hands-over" (hands held one to two inches above the skin) can be employed in specific situations, such as treating a patient with a burn or an infectious disease. "Hands-over" can also be used if the patient is reluctant to be touched. More than one practitioner can treat the patient at a time; these sessions are called team treatments (Baginski & Sharamon 1988; Morris & Morris 1998).

During a session, the patient may feel the transfer of energy as a change in temperature (warm/cold), change in pressure (heavy/light), vibration (tingling, pulsing), or "magnetic" sensation. Following a session, patients generally report feeling a mitigation of stress and anxiety, and an overall feeling of relaxation, inner calm, peace, and balance. Patient also report feeling a reduction in pain. It should be noted that, in certain circumstances, pain may be temporarily intensified (see "Precautions and Contraindications"). After a session, it is recommended that a patient drink water to facilitate the energetic shift. Practitioners typically wash their hands and cleanse the room when treatment is completed.

Reiki is felt to work best when performed on consecutive days. Depending on the nature of the problem, the traditional approach is to provide treatment on three or four consecutive days, with subsequent treatment as indicated (Hurwitz 2001). Cost of a typical session varies from region to region but usually will parallel that of a massage.

Research on the use of Reiki has been conducted in the areas of surgery (Wirth, Richardson & Eidelman 1996), chronic illness (Dresser & Singh 1997), neurology (Kumar & Kurup 2003), stroke rehabilitation (Shiflett et al. 2002), cancer care, cancer pain (Olson & Hanson 1997; Olson, Hanson & Michaud 2003), and mental health (Collinge, Wentworth & Sabo 2005; MacDermott & Epstein; MacDermott & Epstein 2006). One study was undertaken in the voluntary sector (MacDermott & Epstein; MacDermott & Epstein 2006) and two in private health care (Shore 2004).

The professional groups that tended to conduct research on the effects of Reiki were organizations for nurses (Olson K, Hanson J, 1997, 2003) (Olson & Hanson 1997;Olson, Hanson & Michaud 2003), psychologists (Dresser & Singh 1997), mental health professionals (Collinge, Wentworth & Sabo 2005), medics (Kumar & Kurup 2003), rehabilitation professionals (Shiflett, Nayak, Bid, Miles & Agostinelli 2002), and cancer care professionals.

Because of inducing bioenergetic balance and prompt intra/inter/transpersonal openness, in addition to the mentioned studies, several systematic reviews display that Reiki activates inner healing processes (psychoneuroimmunological modulation) and has been useful in recuperation of several physical and psychological problems such as burns, sprains, fracture, and post-operation complications, infections, chronic disease such as asthma, hypertension, diabetes, AIDS, endometriosis, psoriasis, and also depression, anxiety, PTSD, alcoholism, and schizophrenia as well as in controlling symptoms such as pain and fatigue (Baginski & Sharamon 1988; Heron-Marx et al. 2008; Hurwitz 2001; Lee, Pittler & Ernst 2008; Mitchell 1976; Morris & Morris 1998; Vitale 2007).

Reiki not only modulates autonomous nervous system and psychoneuroimmunological state (Mackay, Hansen & McFarlane 2004), but also alters the activity of microbes (Rubik, Brooks & Schwartz 2006).

- **Therapeutic Touch**

It is a "consciously directed process of energy exchange during which the practitioner uses the hands as a focus to facilitate healing" (Nurse Healers—Professional Associates 1992).

The technique was developed in 1972 by Dolore Krieger, PhD, RN, professor of nursing, New York University; and Dora Kunz, a noted healer who worked closely with many physicians and scientists.

Therapeutic touch is included in the nursing curricula of many colleges and universities, recognized by the American Nurses Association, American Holistic Nurses Association, and the National League for Nursing.

Underlying TT is the assumption that humans are open energy fields, constantly interacting with their environment. Symmetrically balanced energy fields are said to create the necessary environment to allow optimization of physical, emotional, and spiritual health. Energy imbalances underlie illness and disease. TT is an intervention by which energy fields are detected and imbalances corrected (O'Mathuna 2000).

In a typical therapeutic session, the patient lies down or sits comfortably, fully clothed but with shoes removed and arms and legs uncrossed, so as not to obstruct the free flow of energy. The practitioner may stand or sit in treating the patient. The practitioner uses four steps: centering, assessing, decongesting the energy field, and balancing the energy field (Hurwitz 2001). Mackey (Mackay, Hansen & McFarlane 2004) celebrated therapeutic touch as "a renewal of the art of nursing."

Following treatment with therapeutic touch, the patients report a reduction in pain, a profound state of relaxation, and a sense of well-being. Studies have indicated that therapeutic touch induces in a profound generalized relaxation response in the patient (Krieger 1979).

Therapeutic touch significantly reduces state and general anxiety (Mehl-Madora 2004). This method also appears to be useful for pain management (Keller & Bzdek 1986), wound healing (Wirth et al. 1993; Wirth, Barrett & Eidelman 1994; Wirth, Richardson & Eidelman 1996), degenerative arthritis (Eckes Peck 1997) and asthma (Krieger 1979), AIDS (Garrard 1995), and stress-induced immunosuppression (Olson & Hanson 1997).

• Healing Touch

Healing touch (HT) is a nursing therapeutic procedure that is deemed a complementary therapy (Dossey et al. 1995). HT is a biofield or energy-based therapy included under the designation of complementary and alternative health care and medical practices (CAM) by the National Health Center for Complementary and Alternative Medicine of the National Institutes of Health.

The principle of the work is that the body is a complex energy system that can be affected by another system to promote well-being (Mentgen 2001). It includes the use of intention and the placement of hands in specific sequences, either above or on the body.

Healing touch was developed in the 1980s by Janet Mentgen, BSN, RN, in Colorado. This method is a combination of several healing techniques such as therapeutic touch, magnetic unruffled, etheric unruffled, relaxation technique, mind clearing, spiral meditation, magnetic pain drain, Hopi Indian technique, wound sealing, leak sealing technique, spinal cleaning, back and heck techniques, chakra spread, chakra connection, full body connection, double hand chakra balance, vertebral spiral technique, "ultrasound" technique, "laser" technique, "chelating" technique, and pyramid technique.

Each of these techniques entails the practitioners to place her/his hands gently on or over his/her body (Hurwitz 2001).

The practitioner employs four steps in his or her treatment of the patient: centering, assessment, selection, and employment of modalities (techniques), and reassessment. HT is taught as a multilevel program with a one-year mentorship that leads to certification.

The use of healing touch is reported to have been successful in the treatment of a number of physical and psychological conditions.

Although many positive results of HT have been reported, none of the findings were conclusive. Many studies were difficult to evaluate accurately, particularly those submitted to the HTI research program, since they lacked vital information, leading to problems with both internal and external validity. As Weymouth and colleagues (Weymouth & Sandberg-Lewis 2000) noted in an assessment of HT research through August 2000, only six of twenty-eight studies surveyed met the criteria for quality research. The reviewer cannot determine whether studies were poorly designed, poorly conducted, or simply poorly reported. One conclusion is that the guidelines for research and reporting are crucial.

In spite of these limitations, studies indicated results in reducing stress, anxiety, and pain; accelerated healing; some improvement in biochemical and physiological markers; and a greater sense of well-being. Participants generally reported improved quality of life physically, emotionally, rationally, and spiritually. If such results recur and are verified, another result might be reduced medical costs for fewer pharmaceuticals, hospital stays, and clinic time. HT might also be another treatment option for nurses to provide safe, noninvasive care to promote healing. Practitioners are encouraged to carry out new research and to assess and administer existing research to test these potential effects.

Some anecdotal reports indicate effectiveness of healing touch in pain control (Diener 2001; Wardell 2000), cancer (Merritt & Randall 2002; Post-White et al. 2003), AIDS (Wheeler-Robins 1999; Wilkinson 2002; Wlkinson 2002), cardiovascular disorders (Arom & MacIntyre 2002; Krucoff et al. 2001), geriatric problems (Gehlhaart & Dail 2000; Wang, Xu, Qian & Shi), depression (Bradway 1998), PTSD (Guevara, Menidas & Suva 2002), and also in wound healing, healing of infections, facilitating lymph drainage, and elimination of toxins from addictive or chemotherapeutic agents (Hover-Kramer 1996; Mentgen 2001; Trapp & Bulbrook 1996a; Trapp & Bulbrook 1996b; Wardell & Weymouth 2004; Wetzel 1993).

- **Polarity Therapy**
  Polarity therapy is a system of bodywork that integrates the holding of pressure points and gentle stretching to balance the energy systems of the body (Ina & Chrisman 2001).

This method works on both integral bioenergy field and special reflecting points and meridians.

It repatterns energy flow in the individual by rebalancing positive and negative charges. The practitioner places finger or whole hand on parts of the client's body of opposite charge for the purpose of facilitating energy, balancing where it is required. Through these contacts, with the help of pressure and rocking movements, energy can reorganize and reorder itself (Watson 1999).

- **Sound, Color, and Light Therapy**

  Owing to its physical and symbolic effects, controlled sensory signaling can be a safe and effective method for psychoneuroimmunological and health behavior changes.

  This therapy is based on using the various vibrations of color, light, or sounds to restore balance.

  Although it is sometimes performed more psychologically as a creative art therapy technique, music therapy is the most common intervention in this domain.

  At the most basic level, music as auditory and tactile stimulation can control attention and promote learning. In particular, if sound (auditory) stimuli are perceived as beautiful, novel, or interesting, they are more likely to capture attention. This has important implications for music therapy (Davis, Thaut & Gfeller 1998).

  Music therapy as a subdiscipline of sound therapy is regarded as a subcategory of energy-based therapy, although it is commonly known as an independent branch of mind-body medicine; especially because of several combinations with other mind-body interventions such as relaxation, guided imagery, and cognitive-behavioral therapies.

  Music therapy is an established allied health profession using music and musical activities to address physical, psychological, cognitive, and social needs of individuals with disabilities (AMTA, 1997). It is the systematic application of music, as directed by the music therapist in a therapeutic environment, to bring about desirable changes in behavior. Such changes enable the individual undergoing therapy to experience a greater understanding of himself and the world about him, thereby achieving a more appropriate adjustment to society (NAMT, 1980).

  Music therapy helps reduce pain, increase immunity, and lower anxiety. Music therapy researches support the effectiveness of music therapy in many areas such as physical rehabilitation, neurological impairments, sensory impairments, substance abuse, geriatric care, psychotherapy, and educational problems (Davis, Thaut & Gfeller 1998; Hanser 2000; Rotan & Ospina-Kammerer 2007).

- **Prayer**

Prayer is a local/nonlocal, intentional healing. Prayer is a request, expression of gratitude, or praise made to another. It is important in the study of prayer that, from a scientific point of view, there need be no presumption about a deity. Of the ten most often utilized alternative treatments in the United States, prayer for self (43 percent) and prayer for others (24.4 percent) are the two most commonly named therapies, and being in a prayer group (9.6 percent) ranks fifth (Barnes et al. 2002).

Several studies divided prayer to personal prayer (local) and intercessory prayer (local/nonlocal) (Hodge 2007). In personal prayer, an individual prays for himself or herself. A considerable amount of research has investigated the effects of personal prayer (Hodge 2007).

Intercessory prayer is commonly defined as prayer offered up for the benefit of another person (Tloczynski & Fritzsch 2002). Intercessory prayer is simply defined as prayer said on behalf of someone else. It could occur in the presence of the other person, as often happens during religious ceremonies such as the laying on of hands, or could be said from a distance, i.e., without the presence of the person who is the object of the prayer (Masters & Spielmans 2007). Typically, either a silent or verbal request is made to God, or some other type of transcendental entity, which the practitioner believes is able to affect change in another person's life (Halperin 2001; Roberts et al. 2009; Targ 2002). Distant intercessory prayer, one of the types of prayer most studied, seems congruent with this requirement in that there is no commonly accepted biomedical explanation for how individuals who are not present with the patient could alter that patient's course of disease or physical condition by offering prayers for healing on the patient's behalf. On the other hand, prayers said by others in the presence or with the knowledge of the patient, or prayers said for oneself, may have as their mechanism of action psychological processes that are at least recognized, if not commonly accepted, by the biomedical community (This is not meant to deny or criticize the fact that believers may attribute the outcomes of prayer to supernatural or divine intervention). These could involve, to name a few, social support, increased hope, or decreased anxiety, all of which are psychological phenomena that likely influence biological processes via recognized psychoneuroimmunological pathways (Masters & Spielmans 2007).

There are some reliable systematic reviews on effectiveness of prayer which represent it as an empirical and effective clinical measure (Bell et al. 2005; Hodge 2007). From a scientific point of view, the study of prayer is the simple exploration of the hypothesis regarding whether this phenomenon described as prayer seems to influence or be associated with a particular result (see Rotan & Ospina-Kammerer 2007; Sierpina & Sierpina 2004).

A large number of laboratory and controlled studies show, in general, that prayer or a prayer-like state of compassion, empathy, and love can bring about healthful changes in many types of living things, from humans to bacteria (Dossey, Keegan, Guzzetta & Kolkmeier 1995; Dossey 1996). From a cognitive perspective, mental focus on improving the health of others during prayer may impact the supplicant by enhancing experienced empathy, increasing supportive relationships, and lessening the internal focus on one's own health or social problems (Masters & Spielmans 2007). A surprisingly high percentage of social workers and other health providers, such as nurses and physicians, appear to use intercessory prayer in their work with clients (Baetz & Toews 2009; Koenig, McCullough & Larson 2001; Masters & Spielmans 2007).

Several meta-analyses indicate effectiveness of distant positive intentionality (prayer) on several clinical situations such as AIDS, cardiac surgery, rheumatoid arthritis, and pregnancy (Benor 2000; Dossey, Keegan, Guzzetta & Kolkmeier 1995; Halperin 2001; Sierpina & Sierpina 2004). Nevertheless, the difficulties of studying prayer in an experimental manner are formidable and require careful attention to the culturally relevant values and practices of those being asked to participate in order to conduct the research in a sensitive and nontrivial manner. It will not be easy, but these studies can also provide important data not obtainable in other ways. For example, a study in which groups are assigned to increased prayer for others versus increased prayer for self conditions would have obvious interpretive power. Conduct of these studies among various samples (e.g., certain denominations, intrinsic versus extrinsic religious orientations, spiritually mature versus spiritually immature, etc.) would further add to the specificity in the literature (Masters & Spielmans, 2007).

Energy Medicine and Health Delivery System

Generally, energy medicine is pivoted on the energetic events and actions as the fundamental and subtle physiopathological level of therapeutic interventions. This energy does not stop at the surface of the skin but extends beyond the body, thereby creating an individual's energy field. The pattern of energy flow through this energy field has an anatomy that includes chakras, meridians, and etheric levels (see: chapter II).

Bioenergy performs two vital functions: (1) In proper balance, energy improves vitality and nourishes the body's cells, rendering them robust and healthy. (2) Energy provides the template upon which the pattern of cellular regeneration is based.

When energy flows freely through and about the body in a poised symmetrical manner, good health can be maintained. When energy flow becomes restricted, disturbed, imbalanced, or asymmetrical, ill health can ensue. Physical trauma, restricted emotions, habitual patterns of negative thought disrupt the free flow of energy, causing energetic imbalance. In the short term, energetic imbalance can decrease vitality, limit resilience, and impair the functioning of cells, tissues, and organs. In the long run, energetic imbalance may damage one's blueprint, disrupting the body's pattern of cellular regeneration, impairing the body's ability to heal, and predisposing an individual to chronic pain and chronic disease.

Energy-based therapeutic modalities involve repatterning of the patient's energy field, restoring balance, and restoring energy flow. Therapeutic touch, healing touch, and Reiki are energetic techniques that have been administered successfully in hospital, hospice, and outpatient settings. Each has been found to accelerate healing, alleviate symptoms, reduce pain, reduce stress and anxiety, induce relaxation, and provide a sense of placidity and well-being. Proved to be effective tools in preventive health measures and disease intervention, energy-based therapeutic modalities are to be used in addition to, not in lieu for, traditional medical therapies (Hurwitz 2001).

Beyond the methodological variations of energy-based therapies, common epistemological principles exist, the basic concepts of which are:

1. Matter-energy-information-consciousness continuum (body-mind-spirit unity)
2. A vibrational cosmology, physiology, psychology
3. Inner healing power
4. Inner health map (bioenergetic blueprint)
5. Bioenergetic transference (induction of a new bioenergetic pattern)
6. Bioenergetic gates (trigger points and/or auras)

In the ensuing chapters, we subject to scrutiny the psychophysical and inter/intra/transpersonal dynamisms of these concepts. Most of the energy-based therapies are classified in energy medicine, and/or mind-body intervention, as complementary therapies but some of them, like acupuncture and homeopathy, are classified under alternative medicine.

In what follows, we discuss the place of energy-based therapies in complementary and alternative medicine (CAM) and then we intend to present an integrative model of bioenergy healing systems.

Energy Medicine and CAM

Vincent and Furnham (1996) maintain that patients in Western countries use the complementary and alternative medicine (CAM) to maintain their health because of the following reasons:

1- They believe that their general health improves.
2- They believe that they would have a more active role in maintaining their health.
3- They believe that oriental treatment methods are respectful of human and emphasis the coordination with oneself, the others, and the universe.

In most countries, the common tendency of supply and demand made the CAM services system as a dish of salad. Although some theoreticians suppose that the "salad model" of CAM services is an appropriate system for democracy and cultural potential development, but this will result in confusion of health system customers (public, local, and professional) and causes many economic, psychological, physical, and moral complications (Bajoghli, Sharifi & Goli 2003).

Diversity of methods and systems of CAM, the differences of CAM and biomedicine in terms of diagnosis and treatment, and the challenges of research methodology of this field makes the integration process philosophically, methodologically, and clinically complex (ibid).

In recent years, different CAM classifications, with different purposes, were proposed by academic and governmental authorities, and also World Health Organization (WHO). Some categorize these approaches into two groups—the complementary treatments that can be used in conjunction with biomedicine, and the alternative treatments that are different from biomedicine with regard of methodology of diagnosis, treatment, and care. Some other institutions organize CAM into methods and modalities, and other classifies them into procedure-based and remedy-based approaches, concerning their different research methodology. Of course, each of these classifications subsumes some subcategories.

A common classification of CAM is as follows:

1- Mind-body interventions (hypnosis, meditation, yoga, music therapy, etc)
2- Alternative medicine systems (ayurveda, traditional Chinese medicine, homeopathy, Unani medicine)
3- Physical and manual treatments (osteopathy, chiropractic, massage therapy, herbal therapy)
4- Nutrition therapy
5- Exercise therapy
6- Energy medicine (Reiki, Qigong, tai chi, etc) (NCCAM; WHO 2001)

Regarding their typical therapeutic and diagnostic methods, some of the energy-based therapies, such as homeopathy and acupuncture, has classically been categorized into different groups.

At first look, various CAM methods seem like a multinational carnival, but from a methodological viewpoint, it is understood that in spite of different historical and philosophical backgrounds as well as different terminology and approaches, they all follow common methodological concepts.

Some of these common principles are as follows:

1- Holistic approach to care and cure.
2- Unity of spirit, mind, and body.
3- Relying on the individual's internal healing power.
4- Individual-oriented treatments (and not disease-oriented).
5- Self-assistance and health behavior modification.
6- Emphasizing on lifestyle and using various life modalities in primary, secondary, and tertiary prevention level.
7- Linkage and unity with nature.
8- Giving importance to education as an essential part of health care.
9- Underscoring the quality of life and spirituality.
10- Focusing on catharsis and healer's wisdom, during acquiring knowledge and professional skills (Bajoghli, Sharifi & Goli 2003).

Energy medicine that is considered as a distinct category of treatment in some CAM classifications comprises all the above-mentioned items in its structure and function.

Energetic approaches, via the mechanisms that would be explained in the following sections, can bring about effective changes in individual's health by means of these energetic fields. However, the effect of cognitive-behavioral changes it can cause is not less than its direct effect (Chen & Turner 2004; Goli 2008).

In addition to the above-mentioned items, which energetic approaches have in common with other CAM methods, theses approaches focus on energetic and spiritual interventions.

Regarding their rapid effect and not needing complex skills, these methods have undergone prominent significant growth in recent years.

Many of these authorities generally consider energy-based therapies as mind-body interventions (Rotan & Ospina-Kammerer 2007), or in a distinct category as energy medicine (e.g., Nield-Anderson & Ameling 2000; Ruhl 2002; van Sell 1996).

In coming parts, the position of energy-based therapies as mind-body interventions and also as clinical approaches to energy medicine and generally as a complementary method of health improvement will be expatiated.

Bioenergy Healing and Mind-Body Medicine

Mind-body medicine focuses on the relationship of brain, mind, body, behavior, and the salient and ways that emotional, social, spiritual, and behavioral factors can directly affect health. It is known as a basic approach that focuses on potentials and abilities of the individual in his/her healing and improves them (Wolsko et al. 2004).

Generally, mind-body interventions include relaxation techniques, hypnosis, visual imagery, meditation, yoga, biofeedback, tai chi, Qigong, Reiki, cognitive-behavioral therapies, and spiritual and autogenic training and prayer (NCCAM).

In other words, mind-body medicine is the study of the way, mental activities exert an influence on health, and using mental interventions can change the content of these mental activities by either reducing stress or affecting cognitions or emotions in order to improve health (Rotan & Ospina-Kammerer 2007). This approach views illness as a chance for personal development that can modulate the lifestyle by passing the health rout.

The history of importance of mind in psychodynamic and treatment of illnesses goes back to ancient traditional oriental therapeutic approaches such as ayurveda medicine, more than two thousand years ago.

Moreover, *Socrates* adverted to the moral and spiritual aspects of healing and believed that the process of treatment is influenced by the interaction of personal and environmental factors.

While the West was dealing with internal relations, and individualistic and analytical tendencies, the East with a holistic view defined the events as a nexus of interactions and human being as a part of the continuum of nature.

One of the first attempts of the modern West to demonstrate the mind-body relations was performed by *Walter Cannon*, 1920.

In his studies, he documented the relations neuroendocrine responses and stress in animals (Cannon 1962). Years later, *Hans Selye* evaluated the effect of stress on health (Selye 1978). Anyhow, technology advancement in medicine and the disease-based paradigms ended up in reductionist and materialistic approaches, and the valuable role of mental factors were neglected.

After World War II, due to researchers' endeavors, new horizons were opened up toward the mind-body relation, and finally mind-body interaction had widely been incorporated within the clinical and research studies by 1960s.

Psychoneuroimmunology and revolutionary findings of *Ader* and *Cohen* came to find a valid basis for explanation of mind-body phenomena (Ader & Cohen 1975; 1982; Ader, Cohen & Felten 1995).

A few decades of mind-body medicine research have provided significant evidence of psychological factor's contribution to various physical diseases such as coronary artery diseases, autoimmune diseases, and cancers. This indicates the importance and efficacy of these factors in clinical fields and treatment of patients. Hence, the mind-body medicine, by providing scientific evidence, has fostered novel potentials in therapeutic interventions to health practitioners.

Regarding the following mechanisms that will be explained in detail, energetic approaches function as mind-body interventions:

a) Cognitive-behavioral changes.
b) Motivating bioenergetic flows by cognitive-behavioral interventions.
c) Direct effect of bioenergetic factors on physical and psychological health (Goli 2008).

Energy-based healing systems as mind-body interventions are focused on how mental activities (e.g., perception) or mind-body interventions (e.g., meditation) may interact with energy and energy systems. Regardless of the type of energy, mind-body medicine is used when we employ any conscious and explicit focus of energy toward healing or preventing a problem (Rotan & Ospina-Kammerer 2007).

Integrative Bioenergetic Health Model

In recent decades, several integrative health models have been proposed on the basis of energy concept, especially in nursing. The concept of energy and vibrational worldview may be useful to organize a more flexible and coherent framework for health theory and practice. Movement, massage, vibrational interventions, as well as nutrition, remedies and even surgery can be considered as energetic repatternings.

In early 70s, Martha Rogers, the pioneer of these movements, proposed an integrative health model on the basis of energetic fields of human and environment that is used as a theoretical framework for environmental sustainability nursing and bioenergy healing systems (Heidt 1981; Quinn 1984).

According to Rogers, energy fields are the basis of understanding life. She believed that human energy fields are non-reducible, non-separable, and multidimensional. She identified these fields with apparent models and characteristics that belong to a continuous whole. This whole body cannot be predicted from its elements (Chang 2001).

Rogers advances a novel model of the individual as a whole and the surrounding energy fields. These fields are in a continuous interaction and move toward the concurrent change processes (Rogers, Kirschenbaum & Henderson 1990; Rogers 1970, 1983, and 1989).

Rogers delineates the human condition based on the following five hypotheses:

1- Wholeness: Human is an integrated whole and is different from and superior to its constituents.
2- Openness: Human and the surrounding environment are continuously exchanging material and energy.
3- Unidirectionality: The life processes exist along an irreversible and parallel manner in a time-space continuum.
4- The life organization space: The order of nature is the best model for lifestyle.
5- Human as an emotional and intellectual being: Human is an amalgamation of thoughts, behaviors, and emotions.

Homodynamic evaluation of Rogers's concepts that are deduced from this conceptual model presents a method to apprehend the uniqueness of human beings and his relation with the immediate environment.

Four concepts of Rogers's homodynamic are as follows:

1- The reciprocity concept: This shows the mutual relationship of the human field and the environment field.
2- The synchrony concept: The human field dynamism at a specific time and space which correlates with the environmental fields at that specific point of time.
3- The helicy concept: It demonstrates the human—environment interactions along a longitudinal helical axis, which are bound by time and space.
4- The resonancy concept: These changes in structure and model of human and environmental fields are made through waves. Human life process includes rhythmical vibrations that swing at different frequencies and are affected by environmental waves.

These concepts which have been revised several times by Rogers (1970, 1983, and 1989) provided a clear and comprehensive framework to elucidate the mind-body (ki) and human-world (Rei) dynamics.

Rogers presents an obvious image of human—environment field unity process through his concepts. The model is the best description to define and comprehend the experiments of Reiki and other bioenergy healing's learners (Whelan & Wishnia 2003).

According to Rogers, health is an indication of field patterning. Hence, an individual or his/her family's health potential can be promoted through deliberate nursing patterning of the environmental field.

To promote health potential, health providers would first appraise manifest behavior patterns of the client, including lifestyle parameters, rhythms and flows of energy, and manifestations of patterning, and then, empowering both healer and healee and accepting diversity as the norm, and viewing change as positive. Subsequently, the healer would become attuned to patterning and use wave modalities for mutual deliberative patterning such as light, color, music, movement, and bioenergy.

Energetic aspect of Rogers's model is clarified in Leddy's human energy model. Leddy (2004) regards the human being (person) as a unitary energy field that is open to and continuously interacting with an environmental energy field. Self-organization distinguishes the human energy field from the environmental field with which it is inextricably merged and entangled. Self-organization is a synthesis of continuity and change, which provides identity while the human evolves toward a sense of integrity, meaning, and purpose in living (Leddy 1998). The human being also possesses awareness, which makes possible intention, the construction of self-identity and meaning, and the ability to influence changes through choice.

The environment is viewed as dynamic, changing through continuous transformation of energy with matter and information. These transformations occur as a web of connectedness in relationships within the self and with the environment, including other humans and/or an "ultimate other." Change is partially unpredictable, but is also influenced by inherent order in the universe, history, pattern, and choice.

Health is the pattern of the whole. This alternating pattern of harmony/dissonance varies over time in quality and intensity.

According to Slater (2000), energetic healing occurs through the medium of energy, "a metaphoric term used to mean the healing that occurs at the quantum and electromagnetic levels of a person, plant, or animal." All matter is energy. "Matter and energy are now known to be interchangeable and interconvertible" (Gerber 1988). Energy varies in quantity and quality (vibration), has polarity (yin and yang), and is arranged in specific patterns.

Energy can be considered as a phenomenon, an actuality or a thing with an inherent ability to change, or as part of a process resulting in change. "In the idea of energy as part of a process, the universe is depicted as mechanistic; things are viewed as particulate, and change comes about from efficient causes. In this view, energy is gained, lost, transferred, or transmitted, and change is the consequence of cause and effect. In the notion of energy as a phenomenon, the universe is portrayed as dynamic; all things are viewed as forming an intricately interwoven whole, and change emerges from the whole. In this attitude, energy is not exchanged, transmitted, lost, or gained; instead, it is transforming or manifesting itself eternally and in unique ways" (Todaro-Franceschi 1999).

Leddy (2006) described several noninvasive therapies as various domains of energetic patterning in "integrative health model."

The theory proposes that nursing interventions to facilitate energy flow, and resonant and harmonious pattern of both client and nurse are accomplished through energetic patterning of human—environmental fields. The six proposed domains of energetic patterning are as follows:

1. *Connecting.* Promotes harmony of energetic patterning.
2. *Coursing.* Reestablishes free movement of energy.
3. *Conveying.* Fosters redirection of energy away from excess to depleted areas.
4. *Converting.* Transforms and augments energy resources.
5. *Conserving.* Reduces energy depletion.
6. *Clearing.* Releases energy tied to old patterns.

In this era, we need more procedural and energetic explanation of life and health phenomena, as the structural and material explanations of biomedicine are not adequate for organizing an integrative human science and managing such a biopsychosociospiritual matrix.

Psychophysical Energy-Based Therapies

In this methodological study, we focus on mind-body energy healing systems, which employ mind-body interventions such as cognitive-behavioral and intentional methods to change the bioenergy healing. Systems such as homeopathy, acupuncture, acupressure, and artificial energy therapies, because of different therapeutic agents and/or procedures, are not discussed, and it may be more appropriate to consider these methods in a distinct category (figure 1.1).

Mind-body coordination methods as yoga, Qigong, tai chi as well as energy psychology manage several parameters such as movement, breathing, mental activities, and ethical and spiritual modalities in order to modify energy systems. Some healing methods such as Reiki, therapeutic touch, healing touch, and polarity therapy directly affect energy system via visualization, bioenergy, and intentionality.

The most restricted interventions and the most expansive domain of effect are observed in intentional healing such as prayer and distance healing techniques (e.g., Reiki II, III). Intentionality is the fundament of every therapeutic intervention, which can be an effective and powerful curative factor if employed consciously and systematically.

Thus, there are several therapeutic variables that are employed in energy-based healing systems including physical (vibrational solutions, artificial energies, tapping, or external pressure), cognitive-behavioral (nutrition, movement, breathing, relaxation, imagery, and other lifestyle modalities), and intentional (meditation, prayer) variables. Each of the energy-based healing systems is applicable to one or more of these healing factors (figure 1.2).

This methodological classification, which is based on distinction of interventional variables and different combinations of these factors, may be useful in integrative medicine programs and research design.

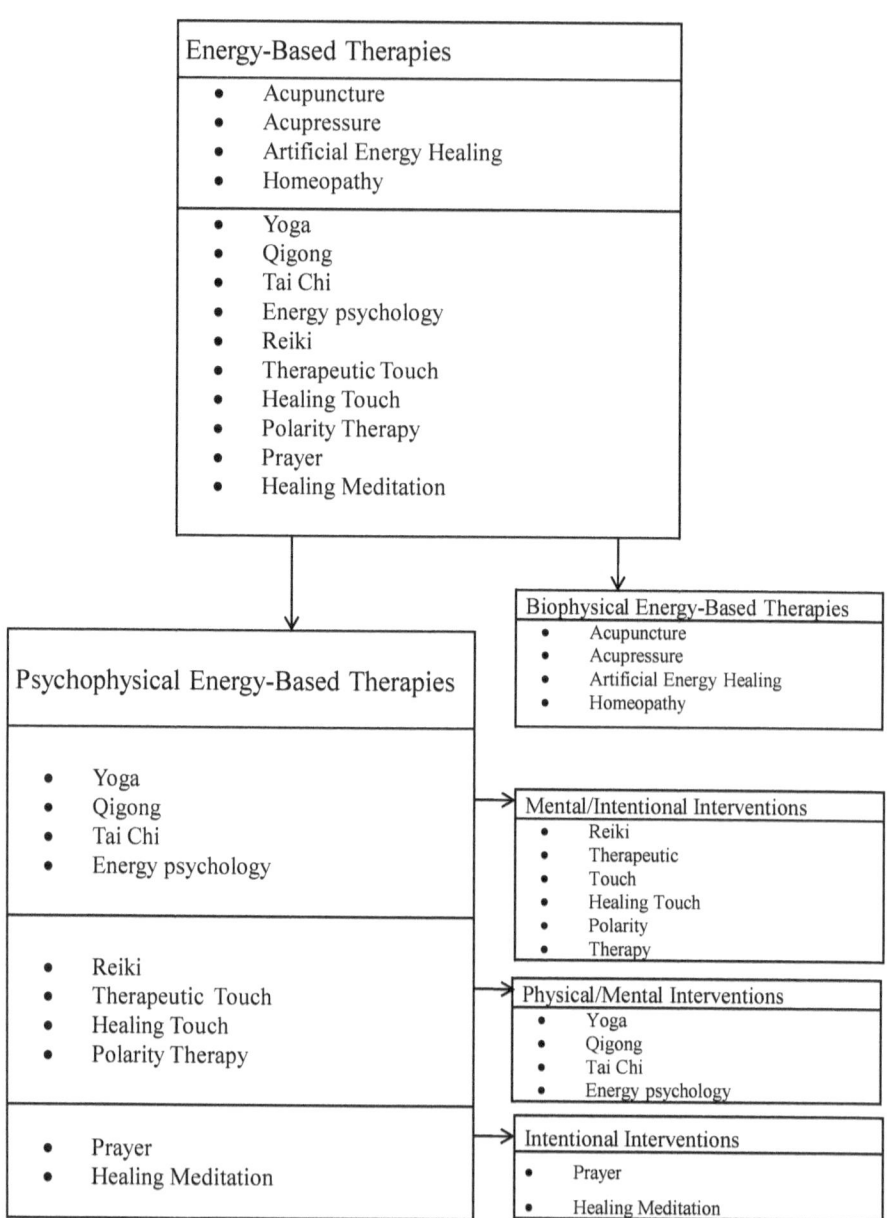

Figure 1.1. Methodological classification of energy-based therapies based upon methods and interventional modalities

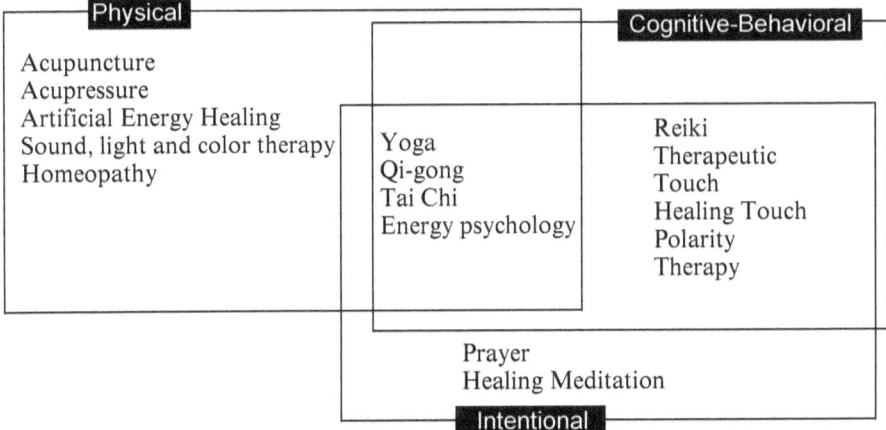

Figure 1.2. Interventional modalities of energy-based therapies

The energy-based therapies which are elaborated on here act on the basis of the mind-body healing system. Both of the interventional modalities and effects are psychophysical.

The psychophysical energy-based therapies rely on the expansion of inter/intra/transpersonal capacities (physical, cognitive-behavioral, and intentional) that are available to assist in the process of self-regulation, integration, and healing.

Mind-body healing is intentional and preferably proactive (not reactive as disease-oriented approaches). Its focus is on personal attitudes and lifestyle, the control factors in the development of stress-related degenerative disorders. The concern here is with psychological development, individuation, personal transformation, and mastery, over the activities of the mind and body to the extent possible (Dacher 2006).

In this essay, mind-body medicine is not only applicable to mind-body healing system, but also to the spiritual healing system.

Spirituality in this model is defined as:

Being aware of the transpersonal world, beyond the intra/interpersonal boundaries, which is characterized by presence (being experience), being-with, egolessness, and/or I—thou relationship.

Meditation and prayer are two methods which relay on the assumption of the transpersonality and the possibilities of the transpersonal experience.

Health, illness, and healing are interpreted as developmental opportunities and processes in mind-body medicine, and the therapeutic procedure is managed in an autonomic and resource-based manner.

Matter, energy, information, and consciousness are in a complex network of interactions and transformations. Thus, intentionality can undermine the deterministic laws of biomedicine. Our intentionality, in itself and/or in the form of belief, behavior, and bioenergetic and psychoneuroimmunological changes, affects the health state of ourselves as well as that of others. The psychophysical energy-based therapies concentrate on development of healthy intentionality awareness of bioenergetic changes and modification of bioenergetic flow and intentional investment, with/without cognitive-behavioral interventions.

Chapter **II**

Vibrational Anatomy

It is thousands of years that human use energy therapy approaches. These methods that are known as the most ancient healing methods exist in different cultures. The idea of energetic relation of each element of the material world with other things existed in different forms in oriental cultures as well as the Western ones (Kohatsu 2002). So it has found great importance in medical anthropology studies and integrative medicine.

In most ancient cultures, this knowledge is transferred orally from spiritual pedagogues to pupils.

As it was mentioned, Reiki means "cosmic energy—vital energy." Reiki is the power that influences the entire material world and consists of the two parts of *Rei* (e.g., the universal and infinite energy aspect) and *Ki* (which is a part of "Rei" and is the vital and individual energy), and "yoga" can be interpreted as the confluence of these two aspects of existence. Based on energy experiments in various Eastern and Western cultures and religions, this power has been designated differently. These names are invested with meaning in the linguistic structure of each culture and, as such, are influenced by specific methodology and philosophy. The Japanese term of *Ki* is *chi* in Chinese, *Prana* in Vedic culture, *Ight* in Christianity, and *Barakat* in Sufism. Belief in this power is called *Mgebe* by African tribes, *Elima* by Nikendo Indian tribes of North America, *Wakan* or *Wakunda* in North America, *Sioux* by North American Indians, *Oki* by Huron Indians, *Orende* by Irox Indians, *Hasina* by Madagascar inhabitants, and finally *mana* as a general term in anthropology. This indicates the spread of this phenomenon in different cultures and also the importance of vital energy in psychological structure and health system of these cultures.

Rooted/entrenched in ancient cultures, energetic approach to health found great importance in thought of contemporary scientists. This energy was defined as *Ian* by Henry Bergson and *Orgon* by Wilhelm Reich in Body Psychology School, which opened up new horizons in the study of this ancient belief. The surface and deep electrical current of the earth that strikes balance in regions with different electrical potentials are called telluric current by Keiser. This energy is vital and universal, similar to Hippocrates, who named this "the healing power of the nature" years ago (Baginski et al. 1997).

Thus, a single phenomenon is named differently owing to methodological, linguistic, philosophical, and ideological limitations of various cultures and has been presented in different traditions and methods.

Do these similarities only signify an archetypal phenomenon and are these data only anthropological facts without any scientific value?

In this study, we do not purport to rake up the old debate of vitalism versus mechanism; we need a synthetic approach to life problem and medicine, and a new viewpoint beyond reductionistic view of mechanism and mythical view of vitalism. Fortunately, though, the organistic and systemic approach to life and health presents such a new viewpoint but because of paradigmatic resistance in biomedicine, it has not yet been approbated established academically and clinically.

In a pragmatic approach, we must recognize every health beliefs, and on the base of their explanatory capabilities, psychosocial effects, and experimental validation, we should utilize and elucidate them.

Vibrational explanation of biopsychosocial phenomena is not too valid, and experimental findings that confirm it are not still so much, but several researches verified the efficacy of energetic interventions on physical and mental states, and its theoretical framework is more appropriate for explanation of human condition and is more coordinated with new-age theories such as quantum physics, systems theory, and postmodern philosophy.

In the subsequent discussions, vibrational anatomy as a health belief system and a biopsychosocial theory is explained and its scientific, psychological, and medical capacities are described briefly.

Vibrational Anatomy: The Scientific Horizon

Physics originated in the sixth century BC in the era of first Greek philosophers in the traditional episteme, in which science, philosophy, and religion were not separated. Hence, the aim of physics was the discovery of the nature, or the basic essence, or of the rudiments of materials. This attitude brings all oriental schools into an interface.

Inclination toward experimental sciences and separation of science from metaphysics and also human basic questions started since the era of Aristotle. After the decline of experimental sciences in the medieval period, in the renaissance by the limitations of the church, a new era was heralded for physicists and a new tendency toward nature started among scientists. Anyhow, this inclination also was based on drastic and strict separation of spirituality and science as well as mind and matter as two different and independent domains of nature and the necessity of reductionistic conception of matter. This Cartesian dichotomy allowed scientists to treat matters as mechanical, inanimate phenomena and see the material world as a huge machine composed of many disparate and diverse parts. Hence, mechanical ideology became rampant (Capra 2000).

Isaac Newton (1642-1727), by presenting the mechanical perspective of phenomena, occasioned an upheaval in the worldview physical ideology of his time. He described atoms as the essential building blocks of the universe, which act on the basis of mechanical laws. In such system, energy is the capacity to perform tasks. Newton's laws of motion are constant, and the universe is described and interpreted on the basis of immutable laws that God has ordained. Anyhow, the limitations of Newton's laws were revealed by field theory of Faraday and Maxwell, soon (ibid).

Faraday and Maxwell, by producing electromagnetic energy via magnetic movement, substituted the concept of "force" with the concept of "field." They demonstrated that the field could be produced from a single force, whether there is another charge in the vicinity or not. This was a profound revolution in human understanding of reality, comprehension of matter, and nature of energy (Ronan 1983).

As such, in the early twentieth century, physicists had two successful sets of laws—Newton's mechanical laws and Maxwell's electromagnetic law. But discovering the atomic and subatomic world disclosed unexpected flaws and defects in the classical hypotheses, which culminated in an essential revision of many fundamental concepts of physics. These discoveries were accompanied by Einstein's theory of relativity, and quantum physics initiated a new age in physics called modern physics.

To give a succinct sketch, theory of relativity deals with the study of phenomena at very high speeds, near or equal to that of light. The quantum theory studies the phenomena at the atomic and subatomic scale.

Einstein believed in the innate coordination of nature and was in pursuit of discovering the unified basis of physics. By developing a common framework for electrodynamics and mechanics as two separated disciplines of classical physics, he took the first steps to reach the unified field theory. This framework is known as the theory of specific relativity.

According to relativity theory, space is not three dimensional and time is the unseparated dimension of it. Concerning this, the tetra-dimensional coordinate system of space-time was defined. The most significant consequence of this framework change is: "Matter is nothing but energy." The relation of the two variables of matter and energy was briefly described in the Einstein's famous equation of $E=mc^2$, in which E, m, and c respectively stand for energy, matter, and speed of light (Capra 2000).

Brogli, one of the followers of Einstein, believed that mass and light are both different forms of energy that can be considered as parts of a wave. This thesis was the commencement of quantum theory (Kohatsu 2002).

The quantum theory concepts, even after being formulated could not be accepted easily. However, they immensely affected the mentality and attitude of physicists. Experiments of Rutherford demonstrated that atoms are not something hard and non-decomposable, but they contain large free spaces in which very tiny particles move. The quantum theory displayed that these particles, contrary to typical materials of classical physics, have a dual nature and are sometimes in form of particles while they demonstrate wave behavior at other times.

On the other hand, all principles of atomic physics are predicated on probability. Occurrence of an atomic event cannot be predicted definitely. Concerning this, it can be concluded that nature is not compromised of separated building blocks, but it is as a subtle tissue or complex connective network among various components of the whole. This is just the way oriental mysticism is accustomed to comprehend the world.

> "Existence of the nature of matters originates from a mutual dependency. They are nothing by themselves."
>
> —Buddha

Vibrational world consist of the waves of probability, not deterministic structures. Chaotic and intentional phenomena can be explained in such a model.

According to Joseph Needham, when the European philosophy was striving to find the reality in essence, oriental philosophy sought it in relation.

But the quantum and relativity theories, in field of natural forces, assume comprehension of subatomic particles' properties possible only in moving, dynamic, practical, mutual, and interactive conditions. Such a conception of the universe in atomic and subatomic physics, and also in Eastern religions, such as Brahmanism is an image of the universe with rhythmic, developing movements with an organic organization. This is an image macro-universe in which everything is dynamic, and flux changing and all static states are nonrealistic principles.

In modern physics, "the forces principle" was superseded by the interactive effects of particles that are carried out by fields. According to Nearing, field is ubiquitous and omnipresent and is never eradicated.

Regarding this, vacuum is not a void, but contains infinite number of particles that indefinitely come into existence and vanish. Particles, in this palpitation of creation and destruction, are the performers of an energy dance. This relentless flow of energies, in which these particles interminably melt into each other in infinite forms and shapes, is a cosmic dance which is reminiscent of the dance of *Shiva* (Capra 2000).

To modern physicists, the Shiva dance is the dance of subatomic events, which is a dance of creation and destruction, omnipresent in the universe.

This incessant rhythmic movement demonstrates that in reality vacuum is a living empty space, in which there is a dynamic relation going on among the particles. Chang Zai (1020-1077), the Chinese sage, describing the findings of physicists, long age, observed:

"The infinity of space, although is called the great empty,
is not completely empty. It is full of *Chi*. In fact, nothing
is empty."

—Chai (1975)

The *chi* or qi energy, which is identical with quantum field, is presumed to be like a thin and incomprehensible shape of material that is present everywhere in the space and can also be condensed in solid materials. Chang Zai also mentions that:

"When the *Chi* energy is condensed, the state and quality of its visibility is in the shape of 'specific materials' and when the *Chi* energy is dispersed, the visibility is lost and shapes are interlaced." (ibid)

Regarding this, the energy is regularly condensed and again dispersed, and during this, all shapes that finally vanish in empty space come into existence. This immense vacuum can be only the *Ki* energy, and this energy cannot be condensed, but to mold new materials and these new materials will not crumble and disintegrate, but to make the immense vacuum emerge again.

Thus, *Ki* energy, akin to quantum field theory, is not only the basic essence of all materialistic items, but also is the outcome of their interaction in waveform.

Rei in Reiki, which originally means movement and flow of all materials and the order of nature in *Rig Veda*, denotes the world to be dynamic. Chinese philosophers such as *Veda* prophets believe the world to be a continuous current of changes (ibid).

This explanation of the *Rei* principle was later deployed to identify the interactive and dynamic effect of all materials and events in the term of *Karma*. As in quantum physics in which material does not have a discrete/isolated meaning and finds its meaning in relation and interaction, so in energy medicine, health and life are expounded on the basis of dynamic relation of *Rei* and *Ki*. As such, energy medicine strives to establish the relationship correctly by means of openness and attunement.

Therefore, in this regard, health means the dynamic flow of *Ki* energy throughout the world that creates and destroys particles and events rhythmically, in harmony with the universal basic vibration.

A reason for medicine, not dealing with such materials and not trying to take account of and the energetic body, is the fact that modern medicine is still based on the Newton's mechanical principles and the Cartesian reductionist logic (Kohatsu 2002) and has not been believed the modern advances of physics. According to Deepak Chopra, medicine still has not still engaged in quantum leap, and the word "quantum" has not found any specific clinical applications. The quantum treatment is getting away the external phenomena and high technologies and moves toward the deepest main core of mind-body medicine. The trend of healing begins from this core. To achieve it and to learn the therapeutic methods, external layers of the body should be passed through and the meeting point of mind and body be reached. This is the point where the role playing of "consciousness" begins (Chopra 1990).

In Dziemidko's words (1999), the modern physics is more compatible with old mystic traditions and provide more appropriate framework to understand traditional healing principles.

Energy medicine is trying to explain the mechanisms of these healing systems by employing attitudes and concepts of modern physics.

As the depth of scientific understanding increases, the physical world reveals a fundamental unity and interconnection that belies a surface appearance of mechanical discreteness and separation. Predating modern physics by many centuries, the basic assumptions underlying healing and medical traditions in most world cultures include an intuitive recognition of physical wholeness or oneness and a view of the world as deeply interconnected (Krippner 1995). Energy-based therapies draw from these traditions, sharing the conviction that the mind can contribute directly to the healing process. While mind and consciousness are not included explicitly in current physical models, a growing number of physicists are seeking ways to do so, motivated in part by a solid body of experimental evidence that human intentions can transcend spatial and temporal barriers (Herbert 1994; Jahn & Dunne 1986).

Energy-based healing models and practices based on intentionality are difficult or impossible to explain within the limits of contemporary paradigmatic understanding. Intercessory prayer, shamanic healing, therapeutic touch, and distant healing all appear to be capable of augmenting and accelerating/expediting the healing process but without any obvious candidate mechanism. Other more conventional practices also are enhanced by slightly understood complements such as the placebo effect or positive thinking. Although underlying mechanisms for the alternative therapies remain elusive, there are some shared elements: The common context includes the disorder prompting concern and the potential structure or information that is required to restore the system. The healing seems specifically to be a function of an intention to heal, and the intentional modalities all share an effort to establish a connection or resonance between healer and healee (Jonas & Crawford 2003).

From a "paninformation point of view" (world as a network of probabilities), matter, energy, mind, and consciousness are different forms of information. Underscoring holistic approaches on intellectuality of vital energy may be an indication of informational view (bottom-up organization) or in other viewpoint an archetype of "pan-semiotic model" (up-bottom organization).

The past twenty years have seen the development of a semiotic and communicational paradigm, largely based on Pierce's semiotic theory (Bier, Wilson, Studt & Shakleton 2002). In this model, human as a part and an aspect of universe is a biosemiotic context and at the same time a sign for the others.

Uexküll and Pauli (1986) explore the semiotic model in relation to system theory in medicine. They explain their systemic medical model as follows:

"Two points are essential for constructing a medical model that does justice to the comprehensive reality of the phenomena:

1. Relationships between significant and significate ("between sign and object") can be found not only in language but also in every area of life. They are the foundation for the bond and interaction of living systems, and they determine the relationship between living systems and their inanimate environment.

2. The relationship between significant and significate is not equivalent to the linking of a cause and an effect.

The signs that make up a given system constitute a code. The knowledge of the code provides access to one sign system and at the same time excludes access to others. Codes establish boundaries that form an "inside" and an "outside" of a domain in which communication is possible by means of this code. The terms "insider" and "outsider" portray this fact.

Codes also play a role in the transmission of information between subsystems of biological systems. The boundaries established by the codes protect living systems from being flooded by foreign signs. The restrictions on the possibilities of living systems as they merge to form a more complex system (on a higher level of integration) can be interpreted as being governed by a new code.

This new awareness has given medicine access to models that no longer start out from the metaphysical supposition of a materialistic and spiritualistic reality (dualism) but rather from the phenomenological descriptions of nature (pluralism)."

Semiotic model of medicine which explores the meaningful communications in living and social systems is an appropriate scientific base for analyzing the energetic body as a biosemiotic matrix and explains the continuity, integrity, and wholeness of mind, body, and nature in the holistic approaches to health. Moreover, the omnipresence of vital energy can be explained with biosemiosis. Intentions, thoughts, emotions, things, and energies are several forms of interpretation of human multidimensional life, an existence with several bodies. In other words, energetic body can be an intermediate vibrational semiotic context between material and mental contexts.

The vibrational anatomy seems more appropriate for explaining hierarchy of life in the basic level (quantum phenomena), and so in a systematic view (pan-semiotic or pan-informatics analysis), than material anatomy that explores static, structural, stabilized, and so visible parts of human machine.

Vibrational Anatomy: The Psychosocial Horizon

If you want to take a high-resolution photo of someone, you will ask him/her to stand in front of you motionless. But most people feel that this is not a real depiction of them. Now, if you want to study the individual more precisely and from different points of view, you have to isolate him from his living and dynamic context more. If you are going to study the components of this isolated body, you may prefer to study the dead body. But are dead bodies the same as living ones? This is a basic question posed by Michel Foucault and reveals the fact that the modern medicine, which is predicated on anatomy and cellular and organic pathology, is a science that comes from the world of death and generalized to living organisms (Foucault 1994).

alternative therapies subject the body to a meticulous analysis in varied manners, wielding intuitive and analogical approaches. However, all these methods, in unison, concur in the existence of diverse vibrational levels and numerous bodies. The material body is at the lowest vibrational level and subtle bodies occupy higher levels of vibration. This model (in various forms) underpins practices as diverse as yoga, kinesiology, reiki, spiritual healing, and acupuncture.

In the subtle body model, subjectivity is understood to be comprising matter-consciousness, usually termed "energy," which is understood to be a constitutive element of mind and the physical body. Moreover, it exceeds the corporeal self into the "space" between self, the other, and the world. This extensive subject is comprised of a number of interpenetrating subtle bodies. The concept of subjectivity is significant because not only it brings a change in the way in which one understands his/her physical constitution—refiguring anatomy as energy—but also changes how an individual is perceived within a broader worldview and to the ethics of relations between individuals in social/political interactions (Johnston & Barcan 2006).

To speak of an individual as comprising of a subtle body is to posit the self as inherently extensive, exposed, and multiple in stark contrast to the bounded singular subject of modernity. In general, the concept of a subtle body presents the subject as comprised of interpenetrating and extensive sheaths of matter-consciousness that extend beyond the physical flesh boundary (the physical body is considered as one body—one sheath of matter-consciousness). Those bodies that do extend beyond the flesh are understood as imperceptible to the five senses but may be perceived by what is generally termed "intuitive" and sometimes "psychic" senses (ibid).

In subtle body schemas, subjectivity is inherently plural—made of multiple bodies. This idea is most clearly present in Eastern conceptualizations of the mind and body, specifically Hindu yoga and Tantra traditions. Similar concepts of subjectivity also exist in many other cultures, for example, indigenous cultures of North America. The number of subtle bodies ascribed to a single individual varies from cultural and religious tradition-to-tradition (Tansley, 1977).

What is similar across traditions, however, is the fundamental concept of matter-consciousness underpinning the idea of a subtle body. The concept embodies a process perspective that views matter and consciousness as ontologically similar.

At the level of the individual, the concept of the subtle body provides an ontological basis for understanding the mind-body interrelation and the expansive effects that alternative healing practices characteristically attribute to even a slight body—mind modification. In a subtle body framework, the mind—matter dichotomy is transformed because both consciousness and physical reality are perceived to be constituted by the same type of "substance" in various styles of manifestation. It is the density or "vibration" of the matter-consciousness that distinguishes the different sheaths of the subtle body, not any ontological difference in substance (or "energy") (Johnston & Barcan 2006).

The concept of subtle body features in alternative healing traditions in different ways, such as the number of bodies and the way energy is to interrelate with its most "dense" form of physical reality. In yogic, tantric, and traditional Chinese medicine anatomy, interrelation with the material body occurs through meridians or pathways (nadi/meridians). In yogic anatomy, different aspects of mind, body, and spirit are known as *kosas* or sheaths, conceivable as conceptually separable but functionally interwoven "bodies." Intervention in one of the necessity means of intervention in others. The underlying belief is that changes in this energy (in this subtle body) at any level, mentally, physically, emotionally, spiritually, will occasion changes to all other aspects of the individual.

Conceptualizations of the *body—mind* as comprised of varieties of force and intensities of "matter-consciousness" are closely linked with Luce Irigaray's (Irigaray 2000) proposition of dual subjectivity (discussed later in more detail) and Gilles Deleuze's and Félix Guattari's (1987) concept of a "body without organs" or "BWO"—an extensive form of becoming that exceeds the organic form. This conceptualization of a "disembodied" body has considerable conceptual resonances with subtle body schemes. It shares with the subtle body aspects of extensity in conceptualizing matter-mind-becoming, presenting subjectivity as unbound by physical form: "It is matter that occupies space to a given degree—to the degree corresponding to the intensities produced . . . and defined by axes and vectors, gradients and thresholds, by dynamic tendencies involving energy transformation and kinetic movements" (Deleuze & Guattari 1987). Further, in a description in *A Thousand Plateaus*, where the BWO is delineated as being constituted by a number of plateaus (1987), the subject becomes a matrix, or stratification, of planes of forces. This idea resonates with the Western adaptation of Hindu subtle body schemes by the modern theosophical society, who present the subtle body as being comprised of seven different bodies that, in turn, are made from matter-consciousness drawn from seven different planes of existence. Deleuze and Guattari (1987) see the BWO as a site of communication between various plateaus (that constitute reality). This makes subjectivity a modality of passage, just as the subtle body is conceived of as consisting of interpenetrating sheaths that, overall, perform a processural bridge between different types or densities of matter-consciousness (different planes of existence).

Similarly, to the BWO, the subtle body posits the individual as radically open, extensive, interconnected, and inherently intersubjective and procedural. It is from such a perspective, where physical-mental-emotional (and spiritual) aspects of the self are understood as inherently interrelated and constitutive, that perspectives on illness emerge in which, for example, gum disease can be linked with procrastination (Hay 1988; Noontil 1994), bone problems with resentment (Noontil 1994), and feelings of imbalance and alienation with blocked energy flow through subtle anatomy networks (Johnston & Barcan 2006).

Vibrational anatomy explores the continuous matter-energy-information-consciousness interactions and interrelationships of organization levels in the life continuum and more appropriate for biopsychosocial health systems.

Vibrational Anatomy: The Medical Horizon

The heritage of years of trying to understand the facts and phenomena with reductionism and inductive methods is the accumulation of valuable data, which not only has not increased our understanding of human condition, but also has increased our confusion and astonishment gradually. According to Einstein, higher precision of information is reached at the cost of getting farther from the reality (Kosko 2001). Mind-body interactions are phenomena have been the object of intense controversy, on which there has been a constant clash of standpoints for years.

To explain mind-body relationship, or to be clear, the mental and the physical, modern medicine is under influence of the Cartesian dualism on one hand that has sent the mind to the human sciences and body to the medical sciences realm. On the other hand, it is influenced by the materialistic model which deems all phenomena explainable by physical mechanisms.

Goodman (1991), by defining a subjective model for mind-body linkage, believes that the common dichotomy between these two is a linguistic issue influenced by symbols and signs, rather than being a natural and inherent matter. Along with it, many scientists of this field and mind philosophers have strived to establish common terminology for describing mental and physical phenomena, or the mechanism that link the nonphysical or symbolic changes to physical changes.

Hence, firstly, we should search for the most neutral words to explain this relationship. Caroline Myss (1997) believes that the only term that does not evoke any religious associations or innate fears, and does not belong to any specific culture, is "energy."

"Energy," as a term, has been used in many applications in psychoanalytical views of *Freud, Reich*, and more recently, *Lacan* and also in transpersonal psychology in defining mind-body interactions. In recent years, by expansion of energy medicine, energetic events have been recognized as the basis of describing the relationship between mental and physical events (Oschman 2000a).

This evidence confirms the perspective of ancient sages who did not separate the mind and the body and typically considered mental and physical events as consequences of individual and cosmic energy changes. Although traditional Chinese medicine and yoga have been more widely deliberated on this issue, all native and ancient traditional systems consider the energy, the force or the nonindividual sense, as the foundation of understanding health and mind-body relationships (Capra 2000; Hurwitz 2001).

The energetic equations are known as the basis for comprehending mind-body interactions and the health and illness, in energy medicine, also the energetic events are not considered as pure electromagnetic changes, but semiotic systems, which are interacting with human as a conscious self-organizing semiotic system. On the base of energetic interactions, mental and physical events can be explain beyond the theoretical entanglements of dualism and materialism, and a proper ground to understand and deal with the human organism would be prepared.

Herein, the question is whether knowledge and theoretical models of modern medicine are in accordance with the monistic prospect of energy-based therapies? Is the continuity of mind and body, human and universe, or Rei and Ki is approved by our modern knowledge?

To answer these questions, we draw on the biopsychosocial model, which is the most comprehensive model in systemic biology and medicine, and there were many plans and challenges in recent three decades to apply it in medicine and especially psychology.

Today, the biopsychosocial model is an outstanding theoretical frame in medicine and psychology which investigates the mind-body relationship. It has been derived from the general theory of systems which was proposed by Von Bertalanffy and Weiss for the first time. Its basic thesis is that the nature is a well-organized continuum and hierarchical system. In this continuum, the larger units with higher complexity level are superior to the smaller ones with lower complexity level. It remarks that nothing is isolated and alone and each system ranging from a molecule to person or culture is influenced by the other systems. All levels of the organization are linked to each other, in a way that any changes in one of them affect the other levels of the organization (see: Engel 1980).

This model, by focusing on mind-body relationships, defines the mental process as an emergent organization in relation with nervous system, which originate from physiologic and chemophysical events but are characterized by their novelty (Goodman 1991).

This view regards mind as an emergent characteristic of the matter, and in spite of being governed by different rules, it is not an independent entity. The difference of mind and matter is in no way similar to the difference of the nonmaterial and the material (Sperry 1969), and human is concerned as a constituent of life continuum and in relationship with other levels of the organization (figure 2.1).

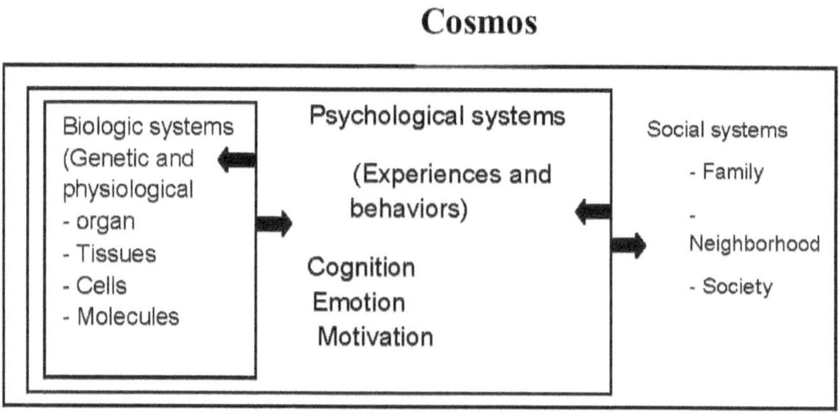

Cosmos

| Biologic systems (Genetic and physiological - organ - Tissues - Cells - Molecules | Psychological systems (Experiences and behaviors) Cognition Emotion Motivation | Social systems - Family - Neighborhood - Society |

Figure 2.1. Interaction of systems in biopsychosocial model (adapted from *Health Psychology*, Sarafino 2005)

The mind-body and human—universe linkage of this philosophical model have some similarities with traditional unitarian approaches of philosophy, mysticism, and medicine. The basic elements of earth, water, air, and fire, the natural qualities, were concerned as the foundation of cosmos and the human, and influence of any of these elements create different humors in geographical places, plants, animals, minerals, and also human.

In traditional worldview, there is a unique foundation to understand human and world, and also mental and physical phenomena. This aspect of the unitarian traditional model is in agreement with biopsychosocial view.

Energy-based methods, by describing the continuity of energetic events, demonstrate the unity of mind-body and human—universe. Hence, in traditional knowledge systems the basic rules of human and nature are the same, and there are no functional boundaries between the events of human and the world.

On the other hand, traditional medicine treatments usually propose ecologic approaches and maintain the dynamic of the systems by changing location, chronobiologic programs, habits, diets, and also proper use of mineral, plants, and animal product.

Traditional physicians have considered this nexus of factors that affect health as the basis of their practice. For instance, in homeopathy it is believed that human—universe linkage is an structural and functional linkage with various mineral and organic materials. Moreover, pathologic and non-pathologic properties of physical and psychological characteristics of the individual have correlation with special effects of a specific substance (Goli 2003a). The energetic and cognitive linkage with universe that *Haneman* reported from *Paracelsus*, and he himself borrowed it from the traditional alchemic medicine, is one of the most common and essential principles of holistic medicine approach (Ronan 1983). This linkage is explained by the fluctuation and dynamic equilibrium of *Yin* and *Yang* in traditional Chinese medicine (Birch 1999), alternations of *Prana* in energy fields, and meridians in yoga (Krishna 2000), and changes of personal energy (*ki*) and its relationship with cosmos energy (*Rei*) in Reiki.

Proposition of life continuum is in common in the biopsychosocial model and holistic approaches, but their differences should not be neglected. It should be noticed that the biopsychosocial model is an approach to organize our vast knowledge of the human organism affairs, which is based on methodological and experimental studies. In an incisive contrast, the holistic medicine concepts are generally predicated on analogic thought archetypal and symbolic rules, and so practice-based experiences. Assuming these two approaches the same, because of their monistic view, culminated in rough comparisons ideological aspects of these holistic approaches, are redolent of the science fiction stories. In contemporary episteme, these approaches are regarded nonscientific, although the tools and research methods of them may be developed some day (Goli 2003a).

Generally, it seems that the systematic view of biopsychosocial theory can function as an appropriate and reliable basis to extend the scope of holistic views and serve as a common language in explaining the theoretical principles of these approaches. Mind-body and man—nature *(ki—Rei)* unity of holistic approaches are evidently based on the hierarchy of explainable systems, and so the need for openness and harmony with the whole is expressly expatiated in this theoretical model.

The communicational structure and vibrational scope of human condition in vibrational anatomy is profoundly similar to hierarchy of life in biopsychosocial model of medicine.

Modern types of energetic approaches, unfortunately, are reduced to techniques and used like pills. In this age, we need a new life world beyond the domination of instrumental rationality in addition to a new body (image) which is not isolated from the other bodies you mean (nature, society) and a new medical model which subsumes several human bodies (physical, energetic, mental and spiritual) (figure 2.2).

Focusing on integrative view in care and cure system and the unity of spirit—mind-body and emphasizing internal healing forces are the prevailing principles in CAM approaches, which discloses their systematic attitude to human, and reveals the contribution of physical, semantic, and energetic aspects to health.

Such view considers health as an interaction of various human systems and gives a comprehensive prospect of it.

This model demonstrates the body-person concept as a tetra-systemic interaction model (Micozzi 2001).

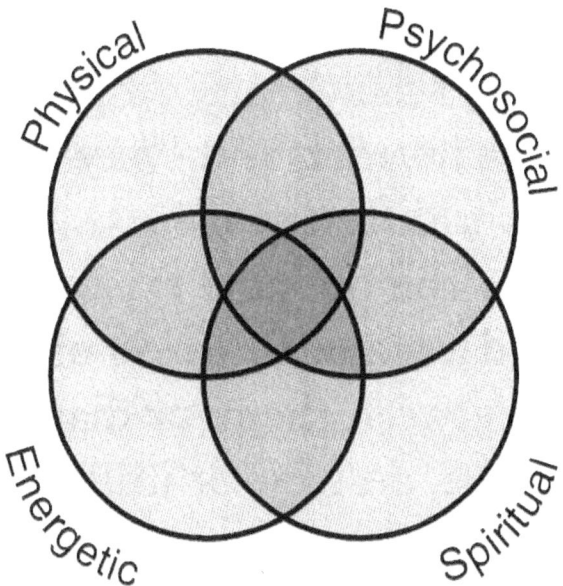

Figure 2.2. Integrative health model. "The interaction of mental, physical, spiritual, and energetic events shape the human organism." (Quoted from Micozzi & Singh 2006, With permission from Elsevire)

This model demonstrates that various therapeutic approaches usually have focused on the study and intervention of just one part of the individual systems and have neglected other aspects.

Biomedicine—by concentrating on chemical, physical, cellular and tissue structures and processes, drug administration, and applying physical interventions—affects the physical system. Even in psychology, the pathological analysis of the body for disorders just lead to medicinal interventions, and less importance is given to other aspects.

Energetic approaches such as acupuncture and Reiki, especially in their Western form, evaluate the energy flow in meridians by energetic analysis of the body and are usually less concerned about other systems.

Shaman healers and spiritual therapists believe in a nonmaterial, invisible body and define the health on the basis of spiritual and parapsychological changes. Most of them maintain that the spiritual forces permeate the physical body, while some others indicate that these forces spread over the physical body, and yet others believe in movement (similar to what occurs during sleep), exorcise (evil spirits), and the loss of the spirit (Eliade 1964; Ingerman 1991).

Psychologists generally deal with the psychological systems and believe that the individual lives in his body and has relations with the surrounding world. Behavior, mind, and emotion are their common terms, and on such grounds, they have organized techniques for therapeutic purposes (Hurwitz 2001).

Bodies are not separate from each other and function as interactive systems that are in relation with and are affected by each other (figure 2.3).

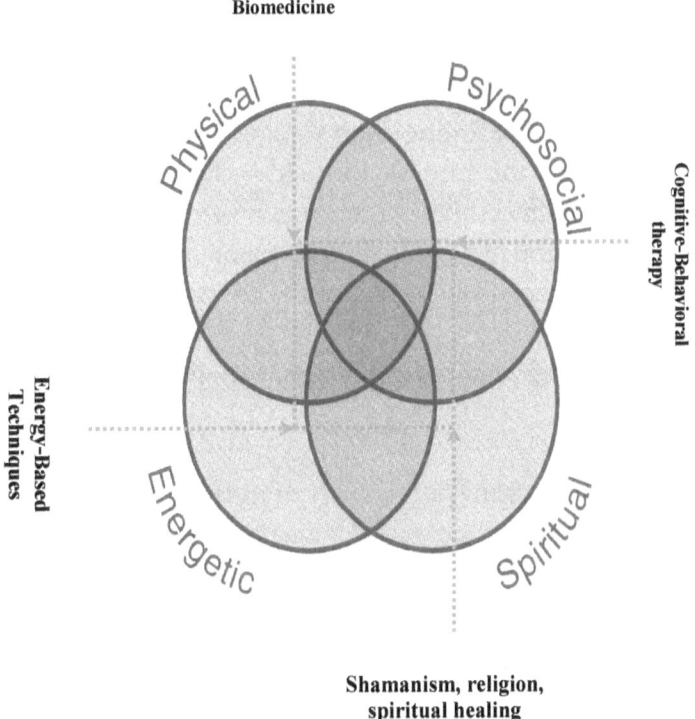

Figure 2.3. Integrative health model; interactions of systems and different gates of interventions.

Anyhow, in traditional methods, there are customs of lifestyle modifications, while in Westernized traditional methods, the special approach and technical aspects are underscored.

On the other hand, there is a growing tendency toward comprehensive and systematic interventions in medicine and psychology and has sought to employ all four approaches integratively to achieve health.

Although in most energetic approaches to health, the main approach is energetic and, of course, in higher levels has the salient characteristics of spiritual healing, yet in its comprehensive forms like yoga it can include the physical and psychological aspects as well.

Vibrational Bodies

Traditionally, in Chinese and Indian tradition, the vibrational anatomy is generally the underpinning understanding physiology and pathology. Some medical anthropologists study this anatomy in the form of cultural body image. But the question that arises is: "Is the energetic body only a part of the Eastern body image?"

On the base of traditional knowledge, we can distinguish three separated forms in the human biofield—chakras (energy centers), meridians (energy meridians), and auras (energy sheaths). Several objective and experimental findings that corroborate some aspects of the hypothesis of traditional energy anatomies are expounded in the chapter on mechanisms.

Leddy (2006) summarized general aspects of human energy field as follows:

- The human organism is a series of interacting multidimensional [interpenetrating, interactive] energy fields (Gerber 1988).
- The energetic network is organized and nourished by "subtle" energetic systems which coordinate the life-force with the body (ibid).
- The physical body is actually a complex network of interwoven energy fields. The cellular matrix of the physical body can be seen as a complex energetic interference pattern (ibid).
- The physical system (nerves, muscles, flesh, and bones) is only one of the several systems which are in dynamic equilibrium. All of these systems are physically superimposed upon one another in the very same space. Bodies of higher energetic frequencies are interconnected and in dynamic equilibrium with the physical body. The difference between physical matter and etheric matter is only a difference of frequency (ibid).
- The higher the frequency of matter, the less dense, or more subtle the matter (ibid).
- The etheric body (vital field), an energetic form that underlies and vivifies all aspects of the physical body, extends one to six inches from the body or two inches on the average (Kunz & Peper 1982).
- The astral (or emotional) body is a subtle substance of even higher energetic frequencies than etheric matter (Kunz & Peper 1982) and extends about eighteen to forty-eight inches beyond the body.

Through thoughts and intentions, the individual emotional field can be stretched to considerable distances, such as ten to fifteen feet. Relaxation tends to expand the field while anxiety tends to constrict the field. Figure 2.4 is a depiction of the human energy fields (ibid: 398-400).

This section of the chapter focuses on explanation of centers, meridians, and sheaths of bioenergetic anatomy. The traditional human field anatomy in some modern versions has been made compatible with biomedicine. Here, we broach both traditional and contemporary practice-based knowledge in this domain.

1. Chakras

The concept of "chakra" stems from the tantric tradition and yoga doctrine. The literal meaning of the term, in Sanskrit, is "wheel" (Kohatsu 2002).

Mind-body interactive processes in yoga are "Pranic events" that fabricate and fortify the subtle body, which consists of three bodies: (qi), mind and wisdom all have imbrications with each other. Prana revives self and the interaction of Prana, and self creates mind and in consequence the practical and cognitive abilities (Rajarshimuni 1999). The pranic interactions flow through different energetic sheaths and organize the vital activities, either physical or cognitive (Goli 2003b).

Prana is comprehensive and eternal; it is actualized via living organisms and is regulated by biological principles. In fact, all living organisms came into existence by commingling of Prana and material, although Prana is not something different from the material and both originate from the basic essence which is called "Cosmos Prana" or "Eternal Prana." Cosmos Prana is a quality similar to mind, hence it is also called "cosmos sense," that is a nonmaterialistic essence, and Prana, as is the mediator between mind and body, is in continuous relation with it (Krishna 2000).

Subtle body has some centers that are called *chakras*, and some meridians connect them and feed all parts of the body with the vital energy *Nadis*. *Nadis* are energy circuits, and their obstruction or any other problem such as malfunction of energy focuses can cause physical, psychological, or spiritual disorders (ibid). In yoga, seven (or eight) principal energy focuses have been identified that are located along the spine and skull and seem to be, in an ascending order, in relation with inferior hypogastric, superior hypogastric, solar, cardiac, cervical, hypothalamus, cerebrum cortex, and neural plexus (Krishna 1972, 1978). In yoga, the physiopathologies of the diseases are mainly described on the basis of fluctuations and disorders of Prana in centers and energy meridians. These energy centers are the coordinators of physical, emotional, mental, and spiritual levels of human organism (figure 2.4).

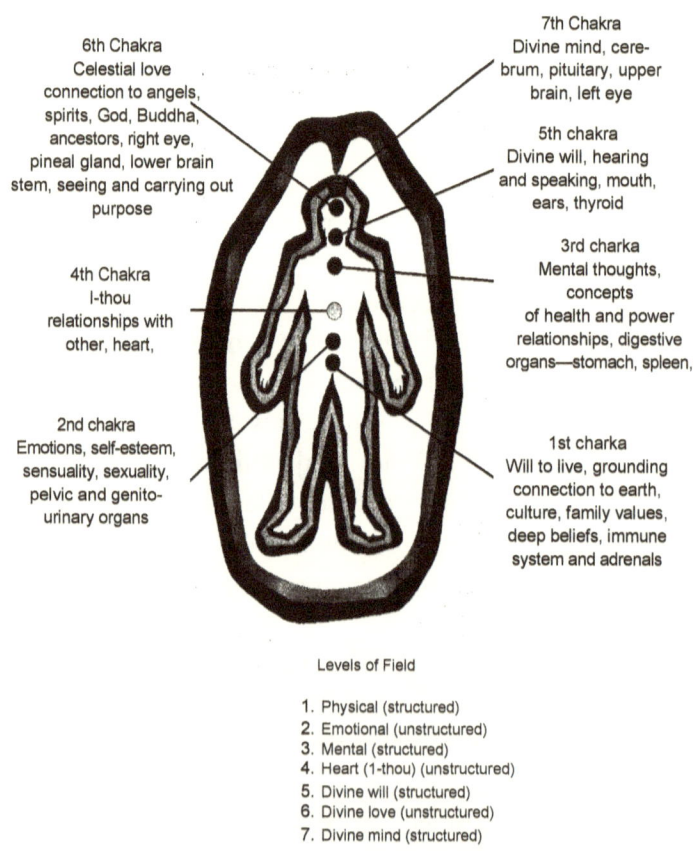

6th Chakra
Celestial love
connection to angels,
spirits, God, Buddha,
ancestors, right eye,
pineal gland, lower brain
stem, seeing and carrying out
purpose

7th Chakra
Divine mind, cere-
brum, pituitary, upper
brain, left eye

5th chakra
Divine will, hearing
and speaking, mouth,
ears, thyroid

4th Chakra
I-thou
relationships with
other, heart,

3rd charka
Mental thoughts,
concepts
of health and power
relationships, digestive
organs—stomach, spleen,

2nd chakra
Emotions, self-esteem,
sensuality, sexuality,
pelvic and genito-
urinary organs

1st charka
Will to live, grounding
connection to earth,
culture, family values,
deep beliefs, immune
system and adrenals

Levels of Field

1. Physical (structured)
2. Emotional (unstructured)
3. Mental (structured)
4. Heart (1-thou) (unstructured)
5. Divine will (structured)
6. Divine love (unstructured)
7. Divine mind (structured)

Figure 2.4. The human energy field according to the experiments of experimental learners and also traditional texts. (Quoted from Stern, J. K., *The path to becoming an energy healer*, nurse practitioner forum 1998: 9, 211. W. B. Saunders With permission from Elsevire).

The researcher Hiroshi Motoyama from Japan discerned that some subjects could consciously project energy through their chakras (Slater 2000). Hunt Valerie at the University of California, Los Angeles, placed electromyographic electrodes on the skin of chakra areas and found regular, high frequency, wavelike electrical signals from hundred to sixteen hundred cycles per second. To mention an instance, the frequency band of brain waves is between one and one hundred cycles per second. It is of great importance to understand that it is the individual's intention to heal and not the expertise of the health-care professional. Every person has a choice of making use of the mental activities for his or her own healing system. Motoyama's findings demonstrate that people can consciously project energy through their chakras and control their own energy (Dossey, Keegan, Guzzetta & Kolkmeier 1995).

Chakras exist within the etheric body. Chakras resemble whirling vortices of subtle energies that "take in" higher energies and transmute them to a utilizable form within the human structure (Gerber 1988). Chakras are distinct vibrations with various frequencies, and each one is affiliated to a specific color, tone, function and organ, and nervous structure is associated with each chakra. Chakras seem to have moment-to-moment responsibility of receiving, processing, transforming, and transmitting energy, information, and emotions that may be stored in the aura. The specific frequency of a particular chakra may modulate a particular emotion, need, drive, and/or organ (Slater 2000).

The chakra system is also an extrasensorial and archetypal phenomenon, which presents the individual's maturity in seven separated psychodynamic stages; each chakra contains metaphorical concepts and specific meanings (Myss 1997) that succinctly describe life spiritual lessons with the seven chakras in the ensuing order:

First chakra (*Muladhara*): Lessons on the physical world.
Second chakra (*Syadhisthana*): Lessons on libido, work, and physical desires.
Third chakra (*Manipura*): Lessons on ego, personality, and self-esteem.
Fourth chakra (*Anahata*): Lessons on love, pardon, and sympathy.
Fifth chakra (*Vishudda*): Lessons on will and self-expression.
Sixth chakra (*Ajna*): Lessons on mind, intuition, insight, and wisdom.
Seventh chakra (*Sahasrara*): Lessons on spirituality.

There are different explanations for the chakra system (Brugh 1979; Campbell 1974).

Figure 2.5 summarizes the chakras and their relationship with the physical body, their cognitive and emotional function, and the diseases related to the malfunction of each.

It is noteworthy that these reasoning are mostly qualitative and pivoted on extrasensory perceptions and clinical experiences of practitioners, rather than being experimentally and systematically tested.

Figure 2.5. Anatomical, Psychological, and Pathological Relations of Chakras

Chakra	Location	Related organs	Mental and emotional state	Related disorders
First Basic chakra *Muladhara*	Base of the spine	Body's fulcrum, base of spinal column, lower extremities, leg skeleton (wrist and lower), rectum, and immune system	Safety and security, will to live, family and group, ability to provide one's life, ability to stand up for oneself, feeling at home and emotional support, social and familial regulations and orders	Chronic lower back pain, sciatica, varicose veins, rectal tumors/cancer, depression, immune disorders, and blood ailments
Second Sex chakra *Swadhisthana*	Pubic area	Sexual organs, colon, lower vertebrae, pelvis, appendix, bladder, hip joint	Emotions, blame and guilt, money and sex, power and control, creativity, ethics and honor in relationships, self-esteem	Chronic lower back pain, sciatica, obstetrical and gynecological problems, pelvic/lower back pain, sexual impotency, and urinary problems.
Third Solar plexus chakra *Manipura*	Solar plexus area	Abdomen, stomach, small intestine, liver, gall bladder, kidneys, pancreas, adrenals, and the middle portion of spinal column	Thoughts, trust, fear, and intimidation, self-esteem, self-confidence, self-respect, care of others, responsibility, decision-making, sensitivity to criticism, and personal honor.	Arthritis, gastric or duodenal ulcers, large and small intestine disorders, pancreatitis, diabetes, indigestion, chronic or acute, anorexia or bulimia, liver dysfunction, hepatitis, and adrenal dysfunction.

Fourth Heart chakra *Anahata*	Center of the chest	Cardiovascular system, lungs, shoulders and arms, ribs, breasts, diaphragm, thymus, and the middle portion of back	Love and hate, I-thou relationships, resentment and bitterness, grief, self-centeredness, loneliness and commitment, forgiveness and compassion, and hope and trust.	Congestive heart failure, myocardial infarction, mitral valve prolapse, cardiomegaly, asthma, allergy, lung cancer, pneumonia, and breast cancer.
Fifth Throat chakra *Vishudda*	Center of throat	Throat, thyroid, trachea, cervical vertebrae, mouth, teeth and gum, esophagus, parathyroid, hypothalamus	Choice and strength of will, personal expression, following one's dream, using personal power to create, addiction, judgment and criticism, faith and knowledge, and the capacity to make decisions.	Raspy throat, chronic sore throats, mouth ulcers, gum difficulties, tempromandibular joint problems, scoliosis, laryngitis, swollen lymphatic glands and thyroid disorders.
Sixth *Ajna*	Between the eyebrows	Brain, nervous system, eyes, ears, nose, pineal body, pituitary	Self-evaluation, truth, celestial love. Intellectual abilities, feelings of adequacy, openness to ideas of others, ability to learn from experiences, and emotional intelligence.	Brain tumor/ hemorrhage/ stroke, neurological disturbances, blindness/ deafness, full spinal difficulties, learning disabilities, and seizures.

Seventh Crown chakra *Sahasrara*	Crown of the head	Muscular system, skeletal system, and skin	Ability to trust life, divine mind, values, ethics, and courage, humanitarianism, selflessness, ability to see larger pattern, faith and inspiration, and spirituality and devotion.	Energetic disorders, philosophical depression, chronic fatigue syndrome, hypersensitivity to light, sound, and other environmental factors.

2. Meridians

The meridian system in the body transports energy in a way an artery transports blood to adjust the metabolism and the cellular change in our bodies. *Meridians* are life forces and affect every physiological system, including the immune and lymphatic systems.

Axial and main energy meridians (Nadis) connect chakras with each other and develop a network of energetic paths that relate the physical and energetic body. Similarities of these paths with tree branches bring the life-tree symbol to our mind, which is used in different cultures (Stein 2000). In Veda tradition, the three meridians or axial paths are called *Kundalini,* which is placed in energetic body and is continued to the end of sacrum. Central path or *sushumna* connects the coronal chakra to the root and makes the terrestrial—extraterrestrial connection possible. In physical body, this path is in relation with spinal shock and central nervous system. The two main paths of *Ida* and *Pingala* moves around *sushumna,* in the opposite direction and are sometimes called *Shakti* and *Shiva* and are mentioned as the paths for directing female and male forces.

These two meridians along with *sushumna* continue their ways helically, conduct, and regulate the energies among chakras. *Ida* is the track of female force and passes in front of the body downward, while *pingala* is male and passes upward along the spinal column (figure 2.6).

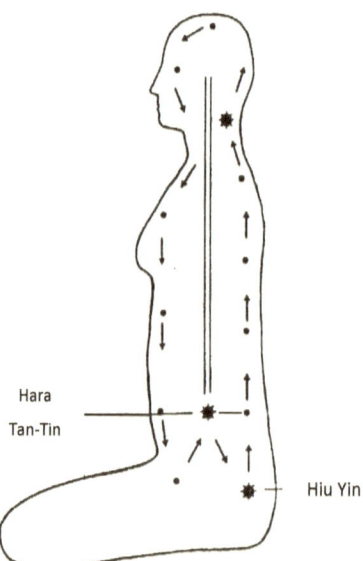

Figure 2.6. Ascending and descending bioenergy arches from traditional viewpoint (Stein 2000)

These three meridians are named differently in China and Japan. The central meridian, regarding its position, is called central path. The bilateral accompanying moving paths are called functional and governing vessels. The female vessel (*Yin*) begins from the lower lip and goes to perineum, the region between anus and genitalia (*Hui Yin*). On the other hand, the governing vessel or male vessel (*Yang*) begins from the Hui Yin point and flows upward along the spinal column and ends at the upper lip (Stein 2000).

In Chinese tradition, there are twelve pairs of meridians that carry human energy. Along the meridian pathways, there are acupuncture points that can be stimulated by pressure, needles, or temperature. Meridians carry the names of the organs. However, they are not always equated with the organ of their name because the Chinese tradition prohibits autopsies. Chinese tradition mostly relied on observations of the meridian's function. For example, the kidney meridian refers to the area of influence of that meridian, not the organ by the same name. Radioactive studies also suggest that the meridian system is separate from the vascular and lymphatic system.

According to acupuncture, meridian system or (meridians or *Jing-luo*) is a unique system consisted of woven strings of a silk tissue. *Jing* and *Luo* mean warp and weft, respectively. Besides, *Jing* is translated into other words such as meridian, meridian, and conduit and *Luo* also translated into connection and network. When these two words are used in companion with each other, they denote the horizontal and vertical strings that are intertwined and function as the paths for passage and transportation of *Ki* or *Chi*, on the surface or in depth of the body. In fact, *Luo* is the branch and tributary of *Jing* (Birch 1999). *Luo* is also divided into smaller branches of *San-luo*. Division of *Jing* into *Luo* and *San-luo* is the same as branching of great arteries into smaller ones and finally capillaries (Wiseman & Ellis 1985) (figure 2.7).

Therefore, meridians are the routes that *Ki* passes through them and regulates *Yin* and *Yang* and control the function of all organs in this manner (Sharifi 2003).

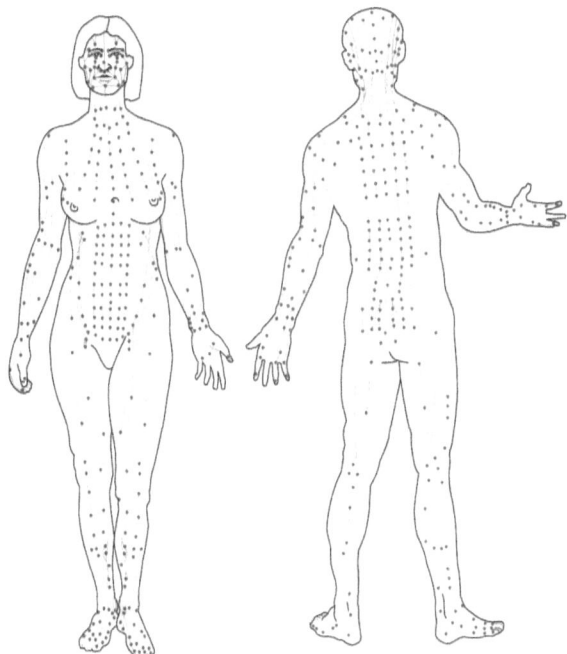

Figure 2.7. Energy meridians (meridians) and their reflective points in acupuncture (quoted from Micozzi, 2006, With permission from Elsevire)

Acupressure and acupuncture techniques work directly with meridians to bring organs into balance. However, in yoga via psychophysical interventions several *Nadis* and *chakras* and finally vital system are balanced. It is hypothesized that any meridian technique is either to calm a hyperalert meridian system or to stimulate a sluggish one (Dossey, Keegan, Guzzetta & Kolkmeier 1995). Meridian-based therapies use pressure points along acupuncture meridians to release negative patterns of emotional and physical response. Psychologists Callahan and Gallo (1998) successfully studied specific acupoints, also called algorithms as described in Gallo (1999).

Meridian network is a biosemiotic analogue system in comparison with digital neural system (see: Oschman 2000a; 2002).

Marciniak believes that the vital energy of *Ki* can be explained based on data (Oschman 2000a). He defined energetic codes of information. Based on this, he found similar models in the information coded in DNA helix and the energetic codes that were stored in meridians and chakras of the body. His hypothesis is based on the codes that are in the form of light strings that our most tiny unconscious data are coded in them. Some energetic exercises unwind these strings the same as denatured DNA helix and decode them. In this way, some states of spiritual awareness and psychological evolutions occur. He believes that healing is the reorganization of this light network.

This hypothesis is compatible with Mollon's theory, which believed the bioenergy field as the source of individual's unconsciousness experiments (Mollon 1991).

We consider the energy medicine's experimental findings about living matrix as an energetic network in the next chapter.

Figure 2.8. Various Meridians and Their Function in Traditional Chinese Medicine (TCM)

Name	Type	Number	Function
Jing Mai	Main meridian	12	Functional Ki flows through them, and acupuncture spots are located on them
Luo Mai	Connecting meridians	15	Alternative meridians for Ki flow
Jing bi	Branching meridians	12	Alternative meridians for Ki flow
Jing jin	Tissue meridians	12	Move, bend, and stretch with muscular system
Qi Jing Mai	Collateral or accessory meridians	8	Function as the reservoir of Ki and regulates its distribution

3. Auras

The *aura*, an atmosphere or luminous glow surrounding something, is complemented by the meridians and by the chakras. The structured layers appear to be standing waves of light patterns with small electrical charges moving along them. The layers are interpenetrating and constantly cross each other, including the physical body. Interestingly, each layer is associated with a chakra. Kunz described the aura as dense light and as "the personal emotional field." Bernnan's description of the aura as layers of magnetic density that surround a physical body and diminish in intensity as one moves further away from subtle energy systems in their body and to influence their healing and to improve their health body resembles a physicist's descriptions of an electromagnetic field (Dossey, Keegan, Guzzetta & Kolkmeier 1995).

Bioenergy fields are not ended within the physical body limitations, but they move inside it, extend beyond it, surround us, and interact with human and nonhuman environmental fields.

Vibrational anatomy does not define a specific border between the body and the soul, and the soul condenses gradually and creates the physical body. Atman, or the individual spirit, interacting with the nature creates the causal body (*Anandamaya* Kosha), and in turn the wisdom body (*Vijnanamaya* Kosha), the mental body (*Manomaya* Kosha), the pranic body (*Pranamaya* Kosha), and the gross body (*Anamaya* Kosha) will be developed, and the borders of spirit and material subtlety overlaps (Rajarshimuni 1999).

Auras are made from energetic layers that are known as subtle body. The closest layer to the physical body is pranic or etheric body, which is the most important body in traditional healing systems, as it is believed to contain a complete blueprint of the body (Kohatsu 2002).

In transpersonal psychology, the vibrational bodies and drawing a matter-energy-mind-consciousness continuum is adapted from yogic tradition. Ken Wilber (1977) in "The spectrum of consciousness" considers the mind—matter continuity in an adjusted form of the traditional vibrational anatomy. He points out the yogic (vedantic) analysis of the human condition into five sheaths on the base of Vedanta philosophy.

The Vedanta psychology of sheaths corresponds very closely with what we have called the spectrum of consciousness, and the sheaths themselves represent different levels of the spectrum. Thus, the outer sheath of the "gross body" corresponds to the ego level, to the self, divided from and therefore a slave to the physical or gross body. The three middle sheaths of the will and the ratiocinative processes (the "subtle body") correspond to the existential level, where the repression of death produces the blind will to live ("vitality sheath") and where the root discriminative processes (the sheaths of discrimination and ratiocination) initiate the hardening of dualisms. The inner sheath of bliss (the "causal body"), wherein man transcends his ego and his physical body, corresponds to the transpersonal bands, and finally the very center, the absolute brahman—atman, corresponds to our "no level" of mind.

Figure 2.9 shows the close similarity between the Vedanta psychology of sheaths and the spectrum of consciousness. Thus, the light corresponds with the level of mind, the doorway corresponds with the existential level, the mirror with the ego level, and so on as indicated in the figure. Figure 2.9 shows the same correspondence, but here the diagram of the spectrum of consciousness is presented with the parallel sheaths of the Vedanta psychology labeled.

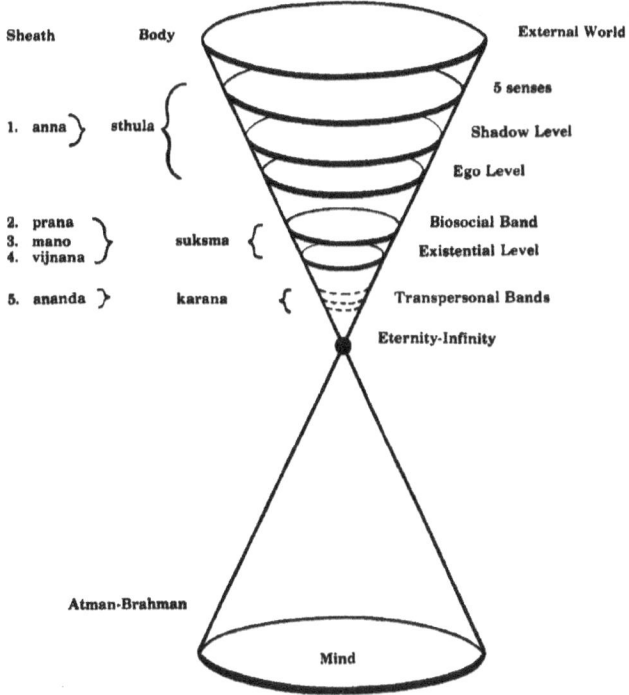

Figure 2.9. The spectrum of consciousness (quoted from Wilber K., 1977, 160)

There are, as one would naturally expect, some differences between the Vedanta psychology of sheaths and our description of the spectrum of consciousness, but in essentials the two are in perfect agreement, reflecting the universal nature of the philosophia perennis, of that "philosophical consensus of universal extent."

Chapter **III**

Vibrational Physiology

Energy field has been a bone of contention among biologists for more risen dogmatic emotions and ideas that originate from the opposition of the "mechanism" and the "vitalism" viewpoints.

According to those who believe in mechanism, life follows physical and chemical rules, and it is fully explained by these rules. Contrary to this viewpoint, through history, vitalists postulated that life cannot be explained by common physical or chemical rules, and a mysterious vital force, independent of the known rules of nature, is active and discriminates living from dead material (Oschman 2000a).

But do we have to choose one of these two methods, the precise analytical but abstract and reductive mechanistic approach or the fuzzy, subjective but holistic vitalistic one? Can a comprehensive, clear view of the human be reached by an objective, deductive method?

A few decades ago, it was not possible, although some attempts were carried out to explain life on the basis of quantum physics (Schrödinger 1967). Moreover, some studies such as H. S. Burrs's experiments on the biological fields and the control of these fields in organogenesis were done (Oschman 2000a; 2002), but until then no independent comprehensive study was conducted. Various laboratory and clinical studies in fields of physics, biology, biochemistry, biophysics, communication, and physiology have been performed, and the science of energy medicine gradually has developed from them. This science studies the energetic events, their vital and therapeutic effect, and the organic continuity of the energetic body.

Research methodology of energy medicine is completely objective and deductive, but is not compatible with the mechanistic attitude. On the other hand, it is not based on vitalistic general view.

In recent years, energy medicine has provided an objective and experimental basis for a comprehensive and organic understanding of the life.

Energy medicine is a procedural and vibrational interpretation of life, which considers psychophysical events in the subatomic level of organization.

The vibrational physiology is a label for introducing energy medicine as a basic science without the topologic and reductionistic assumption of the orthodox physiology. Living matrix, energy-information flows through the intra/inter/transpersonal domain, and upward-down organizations of human organism are basic concepts of the vibrational physiology. In this chapter, we will consider some aspects of the bioenergy physiology.

Energy Medicine

One of the most fundamental common issues of various topics of holistic medicine is the approach to vital force as unitarian factor of mental and physical events (Goli 2003a).

Our understanding of the life essence, by overcoming philosophical and methodological problems and also our deep fear of unknown and invisible nature forces, opens new horizons ahead of us.

For the first time, Maxwell applied the information concept to scientific issues. Thus, the life conceptualization changed into an information system. According to Schrödinger (1967), the living material is an organized system of information and energy. Life is an order that has resulted from the general disorder, and this order is restored by collecting the information from cosmos (Watson 1999). Living organisms, by exchanging free information with cosmic forces and their interactive effects, constitute a unified totality, and human with all his characteristics is a portion of this whole.

By studying this flow of energy and information in human organism, energy medicine presents a new vision to the essence of life, health, and disease.

There is always resistance to new information and ideas, yet after a while, they come to be accepted by the society. This specially is pertinent about the energy medicine with a vague ancient background riddled with conflicts. Hurwitz (2001) conceives of energy medicine as an extensive concept, which is based on the belief that human owns an energy system besides the physical system and the biochemical processes.

In this chapter, we intend to provide concise yet precise answers to the following basic research questions:

a. How bioenergy fields are produced?
b. Through which paths the energy communication is rendered viable possible?
c. Is bioenergy transferrable from one person to another?
d. How does energetic transfer between human and environment occur?
e. Is bioenergy transfer from one place to another place possible?

Bioenergy Generation

Scientific studies have explicated two main mechanisms for generation of electromagnetic energy in the body.

There is substantial evidence that electromagnetic fields generated naturally by the two principal pathways—"piezoelectric effect" and "streaming potentials." These mechanisms play important homeostatic roles such as in bone and other tissues which regulate remodeling and wound healing and even providing a biological basis for successful treatments of fracture non-unions (Bassett 1968 and 1995). There is also an extensive literature on photogenesis of cells and the biological roles of photons in cellular communication (e.g., Pavesi & Fauchet 2008; Shen & Van Wijk 2006)

Piezoelectricity is produced via crystal arrangement of cells and tissues. Our understanding of the crystallinity of biological structures is not correct because of misunderstanding of the crystal definition as a solid structure. Boulingand (1978) indicates that life crystals are sets of long, delicate molecules that are soft and flexible so that they can be called crystals.

Crystalline arrangement in living organism systems is a general rule without any exception. One of the crystal properties, according to physics, is the piezoelectricity. This means that stretching and compression of crystalline arrangements of all body tissues produce electrical fields (figure 3.1).

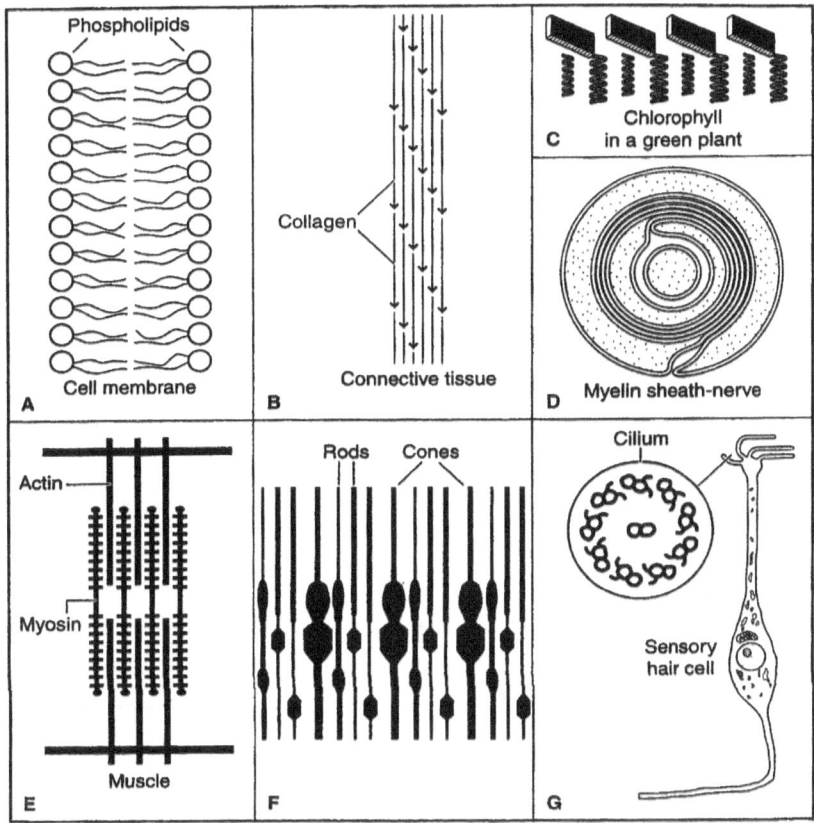

Figure 3.1. Crystalline arrangements in various tissues (quoted from Bassett 1978, With permission from Elsevire)

Physiologists have studied this feature in living tissues such as bone tissue and have measured the resulted electrical field (Oschman 2000a; 2002).

Based on the studies conducted by Bassett (1978), the second energy-generating mechanism in the body is the streaming potentials. In this mechanism, energy is generated via the contact of static electrostatic charge and dynamic charge inside the body. This state is caused by streaming of blood or intercellular fluid through the extracellular matrix and by alterations in cellular shape. These currents can have decreasing or increasing interference with piezoelectric potentials.

Physiological and clinical importance of these electrical fields is to provide compatibility of body with the surrounding environment

(Oschman 1989). These mechanisms are evolutionary valuable for living organisms.

By a brief look at these two energy-generating mechanisms, we discern what a great source of energy flows inside our body. Thousands of streaming potentials and millions of living crystals that produce piezoelectricity are active at each moment. If attenuation and coordination of these forces, which in general condition neutralize each other to a great deal, become possible, then synchronization and control of a great force like laser beam become possible. In the following sections, documents on the possibility of coordination of these forces will be presented.

Intra/Inter/Transpersonal Bioenergy Transference

The idea that science is an activity that gradually and cumulatively progresses toward reaching a correct comprehension of nature and living organism may be somehow misleading. In recent years, we have observed many evolutions in theoretical models and medical scientific findings: But contrary to the abundant evidences on biopsychosocial coherence and a great cluster of facts, which confirm the organistic and systemic approach, biomedicine paradigm persists in its mechanistic and reductionistic approach and try to ignore the anomalous evidences.

Medicine, by overcoming the theoretical and clinical entanglements resulted from the materialistic and dualistic Cartesian attitude, tries to dispense with the ontologic and epistemological isolation and expands its interdisciplinary studies. These changes will provide new potentials for research and clinical experiments and lead to development of a novel paradigm in medicine.

An important evolution in the attitude that can play a very prominent role in these changes is various clinical discoveries that resulted in the discovery of living matrix. Living matrix not only alters our attitude toward the structure of cell and the body, but also reveals the most comprehensive energy—and information-transferring system—a system more comprehensive than the neural and vascular network.

What Is the Living Matrix?

Decades ago, it was believed that cell is only a pocket containing a solution, and its volume is mostly empty. Initial electron microscopic studies bore out these intercellular empty spaces. This space is the place where intercellular materials are either dissolved or floated in it. Furthermore, the cellular metabolism takes place in this space. Accumulation of new information developed the molecular soup model and evoked the idea that this model will soon answer all unresolved problem.

However, physiologists gradually understood that the cell is not just a simple pocket containing a solution and relinquished the model. New preparation methods and novel measurement techniques were employed, and many materials that were thought to be unimportant were evaluated (Oschman 2000a and 2002).

The living matrix includes the extracellular sugar-protein biopolymers or ground substances, the collagens, water molecules, as well as the basement membranes, cytoskeletons, nuclear matrices, and genetic material. Structural continuity between the extracellular, cytoskeletal, and nuclear compartments was recognized and discussed by Hay (1981a and 1981b), Berezney and colleagues (1983), and Oschman (1984), and even earlier by Pischinger and colleagues, beginning in 1975. Historically, the interstitial, cytoplasmic, and nuclear or karyoplasmic elements of this continuous matrix have all been referred to as ground substances (Oschman 1984). Because of their continuity, these matrices form a totally pervasive system, a major organ that reaches into every part, and that forms all of the other tissues and organs. It is the only system that has direct contact with all of the parts of the body (Oshman 2007).

There is no accidental contact between substrate and enzymes or receptors, the way it was thought before, and there is a little water in cellular network in free form (and not bonded) (Ling 1992). It is shown that many enzymes which were thought to be floating in the cell have delicate linkage with intracellular structures and nucleus. Moreover, various studies indicate that cellular matrix is linked with connective tissue or extracellular matrix by transmembrane linkage molecules (figure 3.2).

A

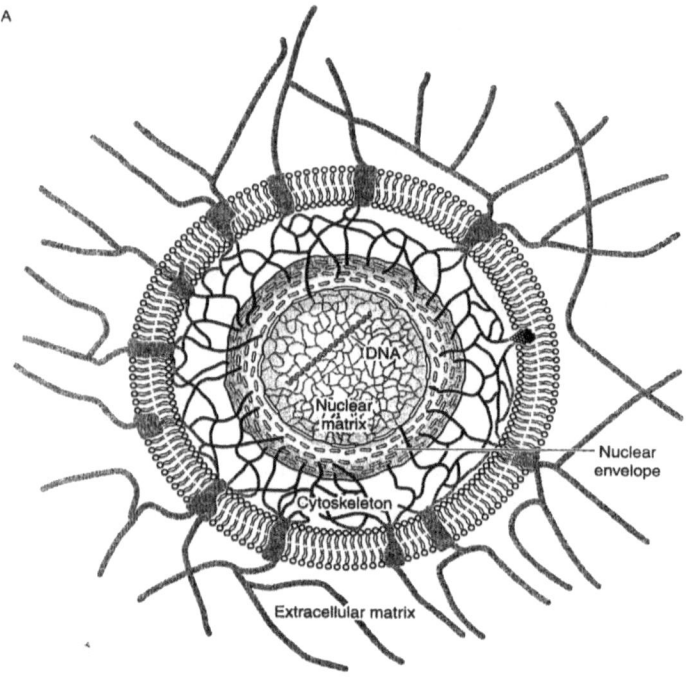

Figure 3.2. Cellular-Extracellular Matrix (Oschman 2000a, With permission from Elsevire)

A group of these transmembrane linking molecules is integrin. Integrin adhere each cell to adjacent cells and the connective tissues. An important study carried out by Wang and colleagues (1993) demonstrated that integrin provides extracellular matrix (mechanical, chemical, and energetic) linkage with cytoskeleton through cellular membrane and acts as atensegrus matrix.

Horwitz (1997) declared that most body functions are regulated by integrin, and this molecule plays the key role in occurrence of arthritis, cardiac diseases, infarction, osteoporosis, and metastasis. In fact, integrin molecule is the focal point of different physiological, biochemical, energetic, and emotional approaches. Moreover, the role of integrin in cells that defend the body against diseases and regenerate the injuries is significant (Lauffenburger & Horwitz 1996).

These findings are important, as making the limits of extracellular, intracellular, and intranucleus environment and the genetic resources fuzzy, contrary to what was thought before (Oschman 2000a).

Thus, the things a body work therapist touches is not just skin, but is an integrated and continuous network that extends to the inner parts of the body (Ellison & Garrod 1984). This continuous connective tissue or cytoskeleton (Oschman 1993) or tissue tensegrus matrix is simply called living matrix (Pienta & Coffey 1991).

Living matrix is an organized, dynamic trans-molecular network that spread throughout body of living organisms and includes nucleus, cellular, and connective tissue matrixes. The nucleolus matrix is surrounded by cellular matrix, while cellular matrix is enclosed by the connective tissue matrix.

Therefore, living matrix is specially homogenized and continuous and provides a consistent continuum. Differences in mechanical, energetic, and functional aspects of the living matrix network makes cells, tissues, or organs different from others. No part or section of this system (living organism) can exist without coordination with other parts, and everything is described in relation with others, and there are numerous various relations at the same time. Oschman (2000a) believes that the defined connecting network that establishes rapid communication between of different parts of a living organism is living matrix.

Pischinger's work (2007) and that of his colleagues demonstrated more than any other that the extracellular matrix is not an inert filler substance or a passive mechanical filter, lying between the capillaries and the cells. Instead, the matrix is a dynamic and vibrant and alive component of the organism with vital roles in the moment-by-moment operations of virtually all physiological processes. Under appropriate conditions, the matrix can react quickly as a unit. Signals can spread virtually instantly throughout the entire intermeshed system in an autocatalytic or chain-reaction manner. The proteoglycans in the ground substance in particular can react to various kinds of stimulation with a form of depolarization that can be rapidly propagated throughout the matrix system. This depolarization resembles the depolarization of a neuron in that it allows transmission of energy and information over great distance.

How does this message transmission system work?

In general, message transmission in living organism occurs in two ways—chemical and energetic. Chemical pathways work by means of hormones, factors, and various intracellular secondary messenger molecules. Energetic pathways are divided into two types of electrical and electronical pathways. Bioelectricity is an important significant phenomenon that results from the movement of ions such as sodium, potassium, chlorine, calcium, and magnesium. This electrical current arises from the great polarity between the two surfaces of the cellular membrane and also the ability of the membrane for alternative polarization and depolarization. This is the way by which messages are transmitted through the nerves. Examples of large magnetic fields in the body are in organs such as heart, retina, muscles, and brain that are produced as a result of the activity of these organs.

Another type of these messages is in form of bioelectronic, which has been studied recently. They are produced as a result of movement of particles smaller than ions. These particles are mainly electrons and protons and also the spaces that electrons are lost in them and are called holes (Oschman 1993; Pienta & Coffey 1991).

According to Ho and Knight (1998), electrical conductance of living matrix proteins or through the proton jump of cellular protein layers and also transmission from interstitial fluid fibers are the two methods of message transmission in solid-state biochemistry. The message transmission mechanism in living organism is described by piezoelectricity phenomenon.

Becker (1991), by discovering a dual nervous system, demonstrated another mechanism of energy transmission in living matrix. He designated that any neural fiber in the body, even in its most tiny branches, is surrounded by one or more perineurial tissue. Concerning this, we have a digital neural network (all or none) and also a perineurial analog network that affects the neural current. The perineurial system is an isolated connective system. As long as the electrochemical digital signal strings pass through neural network, the analogue electrical signal strings pass through perineurial network in parallel. These pathways are sensitive to magnetic fields and seem to be compatible with energy circuits in acupuncture (Ho & Knight 1998; Oschman 1993).

The basis for the above-mentioned study is a magnetic phenomenon called the transverse Hall effect that deals with the semiconductor mechanism. Semiconductors have controllable conductance properties.

This property is used in small electronic instruments such as artificial memories, computers, and amplifiers. Szent-Györgyi (1941a) was the scientist, who discovered the semiconductance property in living matrix. Szent-Györgyi proposed that proteins are semiconductors, and owing to this capacity, are capable of rapid transference of free electrons from place to place within an organism. If a great number of atoms are arranged with regularity in close proximity, as for instance, in a crystal lattice, the terms of the single valency electrons may fuse into common bands. The electrons in this band cease to belong to one or two atoms only and belong to the whole system. A great number of molecules may join to form such energy continua, along which energy, excited electrons, may travel a certain distance. Szent-Györgyi (1988) stated, "Molecules do not have to touch each other to interact. Energy can flow through the electromagnetic field." He continued, "The electromagnetic field, along with water, forms the matrix of life. Water can form structures that transmit energy." The structures he was referring to are the layers of water intimately associated with the surfaces of proteins, DNA, and other molecules in the living matrix. This interfacial water is essential for the conformational stability and functioning of proteins and DNA. Thanks to contemporary research, we can now visualize the way water is organized in relationship to collagen, which is the major protein found in connective tissue (Cameron, Short & Fullerton 2007) and DNA (Brovchenko et al. 2007; Corongiu & Clementi 1981). The importance of this interfacial water cannot be overestimated. Each fiber of the living matrix, both outside and inside cells and nuclei, and the genetic material, is surrounded by an organized layer of water that can serve as a meridian of communication and energy flow. While electrons flow through the protein backbone (electricity), protons flow through the water layer. Mitchell (1976) referred to this proton flow as "proticity." Various degrees of coupling between electron and proton flows are possible. Electrons in semiconductors are fewer in number, but they are very free to move and readily give rise to measureable Hall voltages, even with magnetic fields (Oshman 2007).

Furthermore, Fröhlich (1988) showed that living matrix produce some waves, which moves inside the organism and radiate to the peripheral environment. These waves are insensible. Nonetheless, they produce substantial and significant effects. In addition, as the living material is quite sensitive to these waves and finds its solidarity under their effect, the effects of these waves are not insignificant. These waves are a kind of harmonizing signals for growth, recovery after injury, and organism functions processes. By mediating and modulating the circulation of these waves, complementary medicine systems, as well as classical medicine, will be able to directly influence the defense and regeneration mechanisms (Oschman 2000a).

Continuity of energy and data current exists along with the structural and vibrational continuity, and no changes can be applied in any of these systems unless causing changes in other systems. By presenting the concept of tensegrity system, Donald Ingber (1993 and 1998) demonstrated how these systems interact with each other. The concept was complemented by the paper of Pienta and Coffey (1991): "Coordinated cellular information is transmitted via a tissue tensegrity matrix system."

Therefore, energy and information are transmitted by means of a string of electronic analog signals in a perineurial network, in a continuum of microfilaments, microtubules, and integrins, called living matrix. This information in contradistinction to the digital data is of a less analytic form and is analyzed in the subordinate brain hemisphere (right hemisphere) (Oschman 2000a). In effect, the enhancement of conscious perception of this information results in instinctive abilities and healing capabilities.

Sending and receiving of wave signals that can be sent anywhere without any limitations and signal transmission along the living matrix justifies many clinical and laboratory phenomenon such as energetic healing.

The living matrix and the aforementioned mechanisms can be a cogent answer to those scientists who did not find the above-mentioned pathways in acupuncture and yoga compatible with nervous and vascular networks and, in spite of the clinical efficacy of the accupoints and energy and data pathways, deemed them imaginary and insubstantial.

Matsumoto and Birch (1988) illustrated the pathways related with the acupuncture points and delineated some specific pathways of living matrix (figure 3.3).

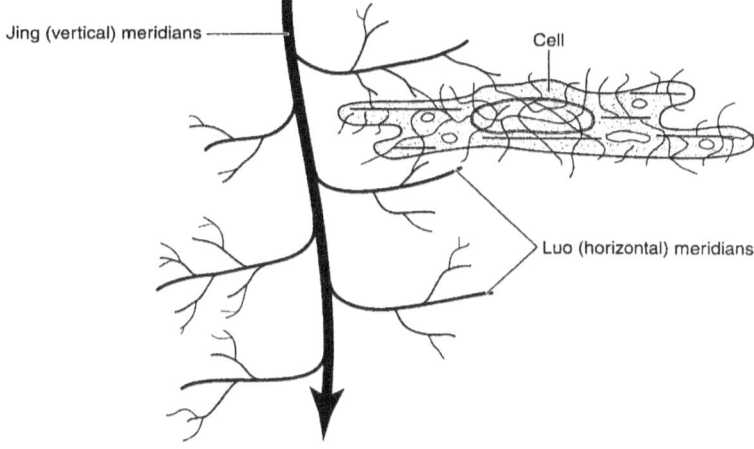

Figure 3.3. A vertical meridian or meridian and its horizontal branches, which are envisioned to extent into every part of the body (quoted from Matsumoto & Brich, 1988, With kind permission from Matsumoto & Brich)

Another question is: Does human being have receptors to receive the intrinsic and environmental vibrational signals? Smith (1994) maintains that electromagnetic signaling can probably play a direct communicating role in living organisms. Lacertians and Epicureans believe that materials are made up of solid and nondegradable units called atoms. The Lacertian biochemistry is premised on the presumption that without any contacts between atoms there will be no intervention. The term of molecular signaling, by studies of Smith and Ben Venist, disclosed an electromagnetic contact. They demonstrated that in living systems each of these signals is an electromagnetic signature that can stimulate different receptors. A molecular signal is presented at the frequency range of 20-20,000 Hz (similar to human auditory range) (Oschman 2000a).

Several researches produce many documents that trigger off the question that whether marked molecules can activate the position of their associated receptor without physical contact. Marked molecules emit frequencies that are synchronous resonated with their receptor and stimulate vibration in it. Ben Vinset suggested that the specific function of biological molecules (such as histamine and adrenalin, etc) as well as antigens, viruses, and bacteria are more a result of electromagnetic interactions than direct contact. Figure 3.4 instances receptors sensitive to electromagnetic signals (ibid).

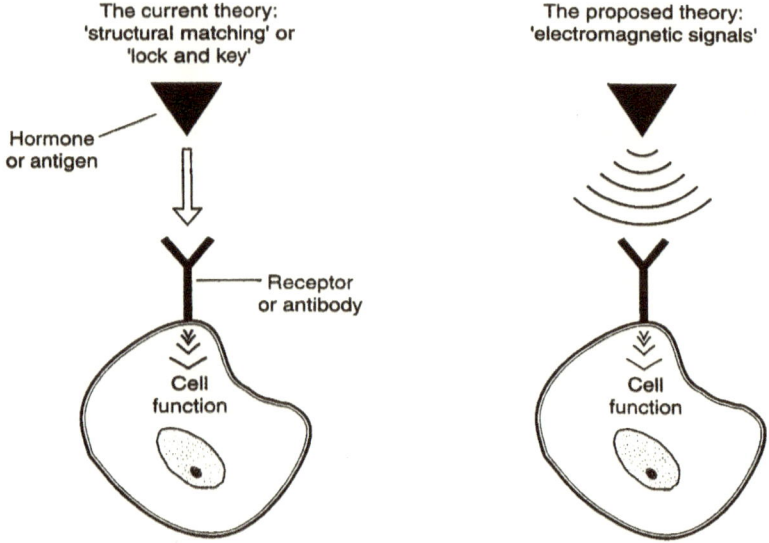

Figure 3.4. Theories of molecular signaling. To the left is the conventional structural matching, or "lock and key," model of biological regulations. The three-dimensional structure of a ligand molecule, such as a hormone, antigen, or other signal molecule, matches the three-dimensional structure of the receptor or antibody. This physical contact activates a particular cell function. To the right is the proposed electromagnetic model. The signal molecule emits an electromagnetic signal (signature) which coresonates with the receptor molecule, thereby activating it and triggering the cell function (after Benveniste 1998).

Concerning all these findings, it can be deduced that the language of communications inside the living organisms is an electromagnetic and energetic language. These findings provide a great clinical and research potential in energetic therapeutic method.

Distance Energy Transfer

Many therapists believe that it is possible to induce therapeutic effect in another place without any objective and materialistic tools. In recent years, many studies have confirmed the possibility of distance healing and its specific healing efficacy (Astin 2000; Crawford, Spparber & Janis 2003; Ernst 2003). However, the mechanism seems to be intricate.

Energy transfer and distance effective interferences can be traced in the principle of synchronicity of Jung (Peat 1987). By presenting this concept, Jung described the reason of simultaneous occurrence of the two events without their causal relation and believed them to result from archetypes or the form or shapes of collective unconscious. Fellows (1997) believe the phenomena of distance energy transfer to be related to the science of radionics and its related techniques.

To explain the distance energy transfer, some researchers pay attention to the documentary characteristics of quantum physics such as quantum nonlocality (e.g., Rohrlich 1983).

The studies carried out by Grinberg-Zylberbaum and colleagues (1992; 1994) on nonlocal interferences demonstrate that when the individuals reach an emotional empathy, then their produced brain patterns become coordinated, and the coordination will not be reduced by applying spatial separation or using electromagnetic hoods. This finding will have many clinical implications, especially in the issue of "rapport." To explain these events, Oschman (2000b) believes that the cause can probably be found in quantum mechanics.

In brief, in classical physics, we learn that waves can interfere with each other. If two waves are of the same frequency and phase, they will have an increasing interference. Otherwise, they will have decreasing interference. There are a combination of frequencies and phases in nature, so many of such interference happen.

In early twentieth century, the quantum mechanics changed the conceptualizing essence of these fields, and after that they were called potentials. Generally, potentials are in two forms—measurable electrical potentials and magnetic vector potential. Measurable potentials have a characteristic; they immediately spread in all places and spaces and are not decreased by distance, while vector potentials have limited speed (Jackson 1975).

In real world, the measurable waves encounter environmental fields, and as a result of the combination, they interfere with each other and cannot continue infinitely. According to Oschman (2000a), these electrical and magnetic fields interfere with organisms and penetrate to the deepest level of cells and tissues.

These findings corroborate the susceptibility of organisms to electromagnetic signals of our surrounding world. However, although the mechanism of this local effect is not obvious and it is inside of our research black box, many clinical studies have confirmed significant nonlocal relationship between the therapist's will and the psychosomatic changes coherent with the will in another place. In spite of using various tools to transform will into an objective action, these studies demonstrated that "intention" can be employed not as a preparation of an action and an intervention, but as an action and intervening factor (e.g., Bell, Suerken, Quardt, Grzywacz, Lang & Arcury 2005; Schlitz 2004).

Concerning this, there is sufficient evidence to understand clinical use of this tremendously extensive network of energy and data that the biomedicine has neglected so far. However, very extensive studies are needed to discover various aspects of it.

Human—environment Energetic Interaction

We, as vibrational organizations, are living in/with an ever-altering complex vibrational environment. Rhythmically changing electric, magnetic, and electromagnetic fields are ubiquitous in our environment. Some of these fields are natural such as terrestrial (magnetic bands, geomagnetic micropulsation, and geopathic stress) or extraterrestrial (solar, lunar, planetary, and celestial cycles), and others are by-products of technology (electrical and electronically devices, communication systems, power distribution networks, and transportation systems).

Earth is a living organism with a very complex and extensive network of matter—energy equations of plants, animals, and human beings. Hence, earth possesses an energetic body that interacts with our matter—energy systems.

The most obvious presentations of this energy include earth magnetic field, gravity, and aurora borealis, which can be measured easily, while there are wide ranges of subtle energies. In the past, these forces were accommodated even in the buildings, and our predecessors believed in a type of harmony between themselves and the surrounding environment (Dziemidko 1999).

Earth magnetic field shifts the tip of needle toward the North Pole. If we observe the same needle under microscope, forward rhythmically oscillating/swaying delicate movements can be seen. Some rhythms are circadian (twenty-four hours), some are slower, and some others are more rapid (in EFL spectrum).

The aforementioned rhythm is called geomagnetic micropulsation. These pulsations are produced by a specific geophysical mechanism: Schumann resonance (Oschman 2000a).

Schumann explained that the atmosphere between the earth surface and ionosphere makes the wave resonating hole. The required energy for Schumann phenomenon is maintained by thunderstorm. In physics term, thunderstorm is a pumper of energy to earth and ionosphere and result in the production of frequency resonance in the range of very rapid waves with a short range of EFL.

In brief, the Schumann resonance phenomenon is triggered by terrestrial activities and changes by extraterrestrial activities that are called in radio terms as frequency modulation (FM).

The produced frequencies in Schumann phenomenon can pass long distances and radiate on and through the body. These frequencies can interfere with biomagnetic waves produced by brain and heart.

Generally, this phenomenon explores the interaction of external fields and biological rhythms (ibid). For instance, there are some similarities between brain alpha waves and Schumann phenomenon that can relate to the compatibility of human organism with this ubiquitous field.

Burr (1972) believes that all living organisms from mouse to human and from seed to tree have energetic fields that can be measured. He described how electrical fields of trees changes with weather condition alterations. Gould (1984), along with the studies of Barr, demonstrated that living organisms could detect severity, polarity, and the direction of earth electrical field. Some evidence indicates that magnetic earth rhythms have critical role in the programming of physiological rhythms (Oschman 2000a).

Some studies indicate that statistically occurrence of some behavioral disorders in human is dependent on the earth magnetic fields or the energy produced by other individuals (Friedman, Becker & Bachman 1965; Perry et al. 1981).

Now, the question is how brain waves are influenced by external fields. Brain waves are not fixed and undergo changes at different moments. Brain pacemakers or rhythm regulator section is located in the inner parts of brain, especially thalamus. This system is called thalamus rhythm generator or pacemaker (Anderson & Anderson 1968).

Destexhe and colleagues (1993) and Wallenstein (1994) defined the cellular principles of rhythm as follows: Calcium ion gradually enters the cortical thalamus neurons, which has the frequency of 1.5-2.8 Hz and triggers off the stimulation and entrainment of produced waves. These waves gradually radiates to higher sections.

Sometimes, production of waves in thalamus is inhibited as a result of excessive amount of calcium ion in cortical section of thalamus. During the silent phase, which lasts five to twenty-five seconds, the brain waves which are called free-run are probably influenced by external fields.

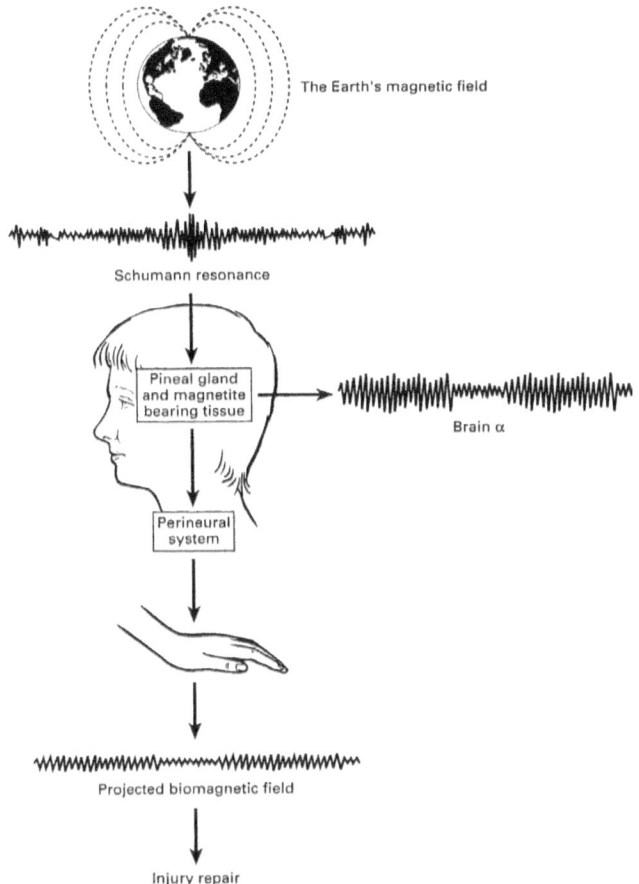

The Earth's magnetic field

Schumann resonance

Pineal gland
and magnetite
bearing tissue

Brain α

Perineural
system

Projected biomagnetic field

Injury repair

Figure 3.5. A summary of the pathways is involved in magnetoreception, the regulation of brain waves and therapeutic waves, and therapeutic emissions from the hands of therapists. Micropulsations of the geomagnetic field, caused by the Schumann resonance, are detected by the pineal and magnetite-bearing tissues associated with the brain. During the 'free-run' period, when the brainwaves are not being entrained by the thalamus, the Schumann resonance can take over as the pacemaker, particularly if the individual is in a relaxed or mediatives state (Schumann signals are thousands of times stronger than brainwaves). The brainwaves regulate the overall tone of the nervous system and the state of consciousness. The electrical currents of the brainwaves are conducted throughout the body by the perineural and vascular systems. The biomagnetic field projected from the hands can be much stronger than the brainwaves (Seto et al 1992) indicating that an amplification of at least 1,000 times takes place somewhere in the body. Alternatively, the body may simply act as an effective antenna or channel for the Schumann micropulsations. The projected fields scan or sweep through the frequencies medical researchers are finding useful for "jump-starting" injury repair in a variety of tissues (quoted from Oschman, 2000a, With permission from Elsevire).

When two objects are similar regarding their natural frequency, without physical contact, they can interact with each other, and their vibrations will be matched or harmonized. This phenomenon, which is called "entrainment" in physics, can describe the mechanism by which body rhythms follow natural (external) rhythms. Figure 3.5 demonstrates the internal pathways that can be affected by external magnetic rhythms when they prompt a reaction in the body.

According to Oschman (1993), earth magnetic fields affect millions of collagen fibers, membranous phospholipids, contractible protein molecules, and even the water accompanying other molecules. Another question that arises is: How biomagnetic waves affect during therapeutic stages?

As it was mentioned, thalamus determines the basic rhythm of the brain. During the free-run stage, there is enough time for the basic rhythm to be influenced by microimpulses of terrestrial and extraterrestrial rhythms. During this stage, we obtain information from our surrounding environment. As you know, the basis of bioenergy-based therapies is transmission of energy to cells and tissues. Chopra (1994) believes that healing flows in a body larger than our body because lesser amount of energy is required for data transmission in that body. In general, the power of a magnetic field depends on finding correlation with a similar rhythm in patients' tissue.

Earth surface, as well as being related to Schumann resonance and very low frequency global waves (that radiates at the approximate speed of light in the atmosphere), is linked with a series of extraterrestrial electromagnetic signals including X-ray and cosmos rays (Volland 1984 and 1995).

Furthermore, subterranean fluid currents such as springs and pipes can produce an energy field that can generate interfering patterns where these currents cross each other. Some of these patterns are beneficial, and some are dangerous. This fact led to the important theory of geopathic stress (Smith & Best 1989).

Von Aschoff (1985) believes that spending long hours or successive days in such areas could affect the communicative energetic systems of the body, impair the immune system, and cause major diseases. Rolf (1962) emphasized the importance of living organisms' relation with great planet fields and presented some methods to adjust the body with the gravity field.

These studies demonstrate that terrestrial and extraterrestrial gravitational and electromagnetic fields, which are sensitive to changes of time and place, can have functional and structural effects on human organism and interfere with our health as a healing or deleterious factor. Identifying these factors and conscious coping with them can have a profound effect on maintenance and improvement of our health. Effects of environmental energetic fields on health:

About 2,500 years ago, for the first time, Hippocrates noted the importance of weather and climate living organisms. In the early twentieth century, Barr and his colleagues discovered the relationship between natural electromagnetic rhythms and living systems. Their studies demonstrated that life on earth is not separate from the rest of the world and is influenced by the forces that are continued along the long distances of the space. Energy fields of human body are inevitably affected by greater fields such as those of stars and other celestial bodies.

The mechanism of this effect includes the interfering pathways. For instance, solar spots and lunar cycle cause changes in ionosphere flows and geophysical fields, which in turn affect our fields.

Arrhenius described the relation of environmental fields and the health (Ward 1972). He concluded from his studies on the cosmos effect on behavior of plants, animals, and human beings that biological rhythms are tightly linked with rhythms and cycles of cosmos forces surrounding the earth. He suggested that the electrical pressure in the air penetrate in biomedicine reactions and influence all living organisms. The importance of information about environmental electromagnetic fields has burgeoned by the increasing of people toward electromagnetic sensitivity (Choy, Monro & Smith 1987; Smith & Best 1989).

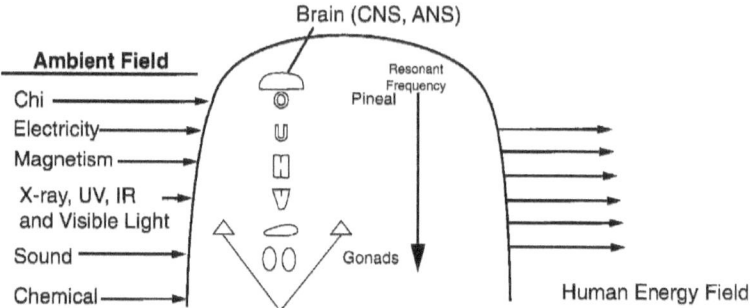

Figure 3.6. Integral human energy field theory. (1) Ambient field impinges upon and resonates with gland transducers, tissues, cells DNA. (2) Human energy field (HEF) is both generated and reflected. (3) HEF interacts with the environment and all living organisms. (4) Chemical reactions to ambient fields affect physiology, emotions, and behavior in an attempt to maintain homeostasis (quoted from Wisneski 1997).

According to Wisneski (1997), endocrine glands, especially pineal gland, act as energy transducers. He adverted to the pineal's role in sustaining our wake/sleep cycle though the rhythmic expression of melatonin has become a matter of pop culture, bandied about the pages of *Time* magazine and *USA Today*. What is less known to the general public—and a large segment of the clinical community—are the other functions of melatonin. Melatonin binds to the benzodiazepine receptor. It promotes the activity of natural killer (NK) cells. It has strong antioxidant properties and reduces aggregation of platelets. In addition to melatonin, the pineal secretes other hormones: arginine vasotocin, LRH (i.e., GnRH), serotonin, norepinephrine, and NAS (N-acetylserotonin). Research suggests that the pineal gland inhibits steroid production, breaking the stress response.

Furthermore, as one of the few loci in the brain that has no blood-brain barrier, the pineal is readily prone to absorb large molecules and the information they contain, without filters. The pineal is also identified as a major source of animal navigational skills, most likely through a direct relationship to the earth's electromagnetic field (EMF), applying an electric coil to a homing pigeon's pineal, thereby shielding it from the lesser signals of the EMF, effectively eliminates the bird's homing ability. Given the pineal's significant role in our reactions to both light and electromagnetic pulses, it seems logical to me to view it as the external/inducer master gland. What is noteworthy is how this role coincides with the historical view of the pineal as the "third eye," the source of intuition, the "eye of the I" that looks out and sees parts of the world that remain hidden to our anatomical vision. The integral human energy field theory is summarized in figure 3.6 as an interactive system. As you see in this diagram, qi emissions which are employed in bioenergy healing are (displayed) showed as an environmental variable.

Although thalamus and pineal body are two electromagnetic gates of the human organism, yet some scientists place emphasis on thalamus and some on pineal gland.

Some people are allergic to electromagnetic fields of 50-60 Hz. These individuals react rapidly when they stay near fluorescent lamps, microwave ovens, refrigerators, and other electrical devices. But just few of the physicians diagnose electromagnetic sensitivity and can treat its symptoms.

Developed countries have established some standards and laws to control electromagnetic contamination, and, fortunately in our country, laws in this field are under development (Oschman 2000a).

Besides the synthetic fields, one of the natural fields is magnetic earth thunders that are caused by solar disturbances and can be so great to affect the behavior physiology and cause some disorders such as cardiovascular diseases (Stoupel et al. 1993 and 1995; Stoupel, Martfel & Rotenberg 1994), seizure and epilepsy attacks (Mikulecky, Moravcikova & Czanner 1996; Persinger 1996), anxiety (Usenko & Panin 1993), depression (Kay 1994), etc. Of course, it should be noted that people show different levels of sensitivity to this signal.

Traditional systems of medical astrology tried to improve health, by culling viable and efficient time and space for healing as well as analogic recognition of effects of categorical environmental fields, especially the changes that are rendered as a result of extraterrestrial great field. It seems that modern medicine, which predicated on the experimental science, should consider such aspects in energetic health.

Attunement Mechanisms

The basic mechanism of Reiki and some of the bioenergy-based therapies is attunement. During this process, the individual acquires the capability of receiving and conducting bioenergy. Most practitioners report experiments such as getting warmth, feeling energy flow in the body, and paresthesia especially in hands during attunement. After meridianing (as an advanced attunement), these experiments are also repeated. Most of these people did not have such experiences before attunement (Stein 2000).

Is there any physical or physiological explanation for these experiments or can they simply be regarded as a hypnotic conditioning? As it was mentioned before, thalamus, with the frequency of 1.5 to 28 oscillations per minute, is the principal electromagnetic pacemaker of brain and the whole body. Regarding this, through the entrainment process thalamus is susceptible other fields.

Wave production by thalamus is stopped frequently and the free-run current starts again (Anderson & Anderson 1968; Wallenstein 1994).

During the free-run stage, we have direct link with our environment. This is probably an adjustment mechanism to be affected by terrestrial—extraterrestrial waves as well as surrounding biological fields alternatively. Evidently, because of the physical, psychological, and energetic stresses, some disorders will occur in energetic fields. These disorders sometimes may permanently remain in the organism and give rise to symptoms and diseases.

It seems that these short attunement courses, which occur during the free-run course, are not sufficient for readjustment of electromagnetic chaos of the system, and longer courses are probably needed. Perhaps to induce the health frequency to the system, more powerful environmental energy is needed. Attunement with the Schumann resonance, which is an electromagnetic bubble within which life has evolved and developed inside it and is quite similar to brain alpha waves in shape and domain of the waves, can lead to autonomous system and hemodynamic stability, and the individual experiences tranquility.

It seems that in deep tranquility and passive concentration, which are developed during relaxation, meditation, and also attunement process, alpha waves extend as a result of prolonged free-run phase. Besides, the result of healing and euphoric experiments during this state is that the system has enough time to reorganize itself energetically. When an individual is under the influence of radiations of an electromagnetic field of an expert bioenergy therapist (7-30 Hz), the attunement can have deeper effects. During the resonance process, the blueprint of a healthy organism is transmitted to the individual, which in turn enables the individual to repeat the experiment solely (Goli 2008).

Oschman (2002) believes that human body has an aqueous system, which is a real receptor for the field that is present in the world. This is the aqueous system that absorbs the waves, and considering the fact that water has a memory just like a homeopathic solution, it saves energy in itself. The process of memorization can be considered as another mechanism of attunement.

Considering what was mentioned above, attunement with the surrounding world can also occur during openness of relaxation. However, attunements in Reiki find direct, transpersonal, and more complex aspects, and energy and information flows from the expert practitioner toward the learner or the patient. This process can result in openness and also expansion capacity of individual's bioenergy meridians and consequently attunement.

In most of bioenergy-based therapies, such as Qigong and therapeutic touch, attunement occurs implicitly during openness and bioenergy trainings. In this experiment, healer plays the role of a facilitator and increasing transformator, which refines the environmental waves and transfers them to the individual.

As it can be deduced from the previous experiments of energy therapists and patients, dependent on the type and stage of attunement, various filters are placed against the current that lead to formation of different experimental models from this selective energy and information current.

Attunement probably can be mentioned as the most comprehensive term of Reiki, since the ultimate goal of the approach is to provide attunement of Rei and Ki. Nevertheless, this is the goal of all energetic approaches and in general the goal of all holistic and human-oriented approaches to health.

Parsimory principle, as advanced here, is one of the most decisive factors which plays a pivotal role in the methodology. Hence the simpler the field and the more relieved of dispensable and disruptive elements, the higher the possibility of achieving the altimate goal, which is the co-ordination of all levels of human life. Adding ideological and shamanistic elements can easily cause a deviation in the process and will lead the individual to abnormal or sometimes paranormal and, of course, useless experiments rather than promoting the individual to higher levels of health and wisdom (Goli 2008).

The important issues in this process are openness of the practitioner as well as the receiver and not forgetting the main goal or the experiment of healing presence as unity and attunement with himself/herself, others, and the universe. The process of treatment and healing is secondary to this transcendental goal.

Nonanalytical Methods with an Analytical Basis

The basic studies that are summarized in figure 3.8 and also many other studies, which were carried out in energy medicine in recent years, have often verified the theories of energetic approaches to health.

Figure 3.7. Outline of Some of the Fundamental Studies on
Energetic Health Approaches

Energy production mechanism	- Piezoelectricity - Streaming of potentials	- (Bouligand 1978) - (Bassett 1995) - (Bassett 1968) - (MacGinitie 1995)
Energy transfer mechanism in the body	- Integrant linking molecules - Living, cellular, intracellular, . . . matrix - Chemical pathways - Energetic, electrical, and electronic pathways - Perineurial network - Hall transfer effect (semi-conductance mechanism) - Tensegrous systems	- (Becker 1991) - (Ho & Knight 1998) - (Horwitz 1997) - (Ingber 1998) - (Mitchell 1976) - (Pienta & Coffey 1991) - (Szent-Gyorgyi 1941b)
Energy transfer mechanism to the body	- Evoked fields - Hot qi/cold qi - Electromagnetic signaling - Energy cycles	- (Chien et al. 1991a) - (Oschman & Oschman 1994) - (Chien et al. 1991b) - (Oschman 1993) - (Schwartz et al. 1991) - (Zimmerman 1990)
Energetic interaction of human—environment mechanism	- Schumann resonance - Thalamus pacemaking - Entrainment - Pineal rhythm	- (Schumann & Knight 1954) - (Wisneski 1997) - (Oschman 2000b) - (Anderson & Anderson 1968) (Oschman 2002)
Distance energy transfer mechanism	- Interfering pathways - Jung's synchronicity principle - Nonlocal quantum	- (Peat 1987) - (Rohrlich 1983)

Identifying the fields and energy pathways and their vital role provide a deep understanding of these approaches. It seems that the highly complex and widespread network of living matrix along with the vasculature network, which is oriented toward homeostasis and stabilization of internal environment, and also the nervous system, besides playing the homeostatic role, providing analytical and conceptualized basis. Living matrix in addition to coordinating of homeostatic activities can develop personal experience and transpersonal perception (Goli 2008).

As Becker (1991) mentioned, the flow of energy and information in right hemisphere usually processes via the perineurial tissue, which is a current of analogue signals, and its result are intuition and personal perceptions.

Orientation of all energetic approaches to intra/inter/transpersonal experiments as well as intuitive perceptions, which occurs frequently in bioenergy healing and training, is probably because of extention of consciousness to right hemisphere perceptions. So it is natural that although these approaches have a scientific basis, they have remained nonanalytical and qualitative (Goli 2008).

Presence of measurement techniques to evaluate the changes in energy fields and a relative understanding of the production, leading and also their effect mechanisms, provided the conditions to integrate these methods in health services system and referral system. There is only a need to prepare organized educational programs for physicians and nurses and also organize bioenergy and also making references of the field accessible to them. To achieve this, practitioners should have a scientific and systematic apprehension of their therapeutic approach and can separate the effective elements from the cultural, ideological, and taste aspects. A postmodern health system should also have a scientific attitude and be free from bias resulting from the biomedicine patterns to be able to take the advantage of the great potentials of energetic approach to health.

Chapter *IV*

Dynamics and Kinetics of Biofield

In pharmacology, the interactions between a drug and the biologic system are divided into two categories: pharmacodynamic interactions, the effect of the drug on the body, and pharmacokinetic interactions, the way in which the body handles the drug. In this part of our study, employ such a classification to clarify the interactions between human condition (as body, mind, and consciousness) and intentional bioenergetic interventions; "intentional" because all of the bioenergy-based interventions prepare, project, activate, and/or absorb the biofields intentionally.

Although the energy-information flow is vitally continuous and is in perpetual commutation between the internal and external spaces, intentionality is the main assumption of healing process that works as modulator of the disturbed biofield to an organized healthy pattern.

Contrary to behavioristic viewpoint, conscious intentionality can function as free will, and physical and behavioral determinism cannot explain intentional phenomena. Acceptance of this autonomic role is the fundamental rule of the healing systems.

"*Qi*" (*Ki*) in the oriental healing systems virtually means intentional biofield that can be sended and/or received intentionally, but *Rei* is not dependent on the human will. It is omnipresent and omnipotent, and we can only be exposed or foreclosed to it.

By this, I mean adopting "Qidynamics" and "Qikinetics" for explaining the interactions of international bioenergetic interventions and human biofield.

Qidynamics concerns studies on the effects of intentional bioenergy modalities on the human organism and the pathways through which the basic physiological processes are modulated directly. But Qikinetics focuses on the systemic responses to intentional bioenergy modalities such as cognitive, emotional, behavioral, spiritual, and psychoneuroimmunological consequences of the bioenergetic interventions.

In Qikinetics, our field of study is contained all of specific and nonspecific effects of interventions because of the clinical and qualitative nature of this domain. But in Qidynamics, we consider only specific effects and quantitative, objective, and experimental aspects of bioenergetic interventions. Thus, a Qikinetics consideration is more similar to a real bioenergy healing experience. It will be more complex, integrative, and multidisciplinary but of less specificity and precision. Nevertheless, these two approaches can complement each other.

In this chapter, we recapitulate Qidynamic and Qikinetic aspects of bioenergy-based therapies as an analytic model for differentiating various healing pathways that are involved in healing process.

This analysis, like every categorization, cannot accommodate and investigate into all of the dynamisms of such a complex phenomena as bioenergy healing. But it may be useful for recognizing various healing mechanisms and so designing more appropriate interventions and studies.

Qidynamics	Qikinetics
Quantitative analysis	Quantitative/qualitative analysis
Objective issues	Subjective/objective issues
Reductionistic approach	Systemic approach
Specific effects	Specific/nonspecific effects
More experimental	More clinical
On the base of linear causality	On the base of circular causality
Disease-oriented	Person-oriented

Figure 4.1. A methodological comparison between Qidynamic and Qikinetic studies on intentional bioenergetic interventions

Qidynamic Mechanisms

Several studies have displayed *in vitro* and *in vivo* effects of intentional bioenergy interventions, and various hypotheses and theories have been considered in this domain.

In vitro studies of biofield therapies are able to be performed in tightly controlled environments that minimize confounding variables such as the power of suggestion. A large number of in vitro studies are reported in the Chinese literature, almost all of which are positive but were judged as being of poor quality (Jonas & Crawford 2003). Recently, a small number of well-designed *in vitro* investigations have been reported in peer-reviewed journals, with mixed results. Shah and colleagues (1999) were unable to find statistically significant growth inhibition of cultured cancer cells following biofield treatments by a Yuangi medicine healer. Likewise, Zacharias and colleagues (2005) found no evidence that biofield treatments by three different biofield practitioners could influence the viability of cultured human cancer cells. In contrast, Ohnishi and colleagues (2005) reported that biofield treatments in the form of external bioenergy emission can increase intracellular calcium concentrations, which may serve as an objective measure for assessing and validating bioenergetic effects. Positive results from well-controlled studies were reported in which Reiki practitioners were apparently able to affect the growth of heat-shocked bacteria. These authors attribute the success of their experimental model to the incorporation of a healing context. This context was provided in such a way that practitioners were engaged in actual healing interventions, and the cell cultures were located next to a patient so as to be exposed to collateral biofield energy.

Almost all specialists concur that reported effects of biofield therapies on cultured cells are difficult to evaluate because they are small in magnitude and are highly variable. One striking exception is a report from researchers at the University of Oklahoma with an international group of collaborators including coauthors from the University of Sherbrooke, Harvard Medical School, and The National Institutes of Health (Yan et al. 2004). This group tested whether treatments by a well-known Qigong practitioner can protect cultured rat brain cells from cell death caused by oxidative stress in the form of exposure to hydrogen peroxide (H_2O_2).

Qigong treatments had a profoundly protective effect on H_2O_2-induced cell death, along with stimulation of cell survival enzymes and upregulation of gene expression for a cellular growth factor. The report from the University of Oklahoma has the potential to become a landmark study in the field, considering the magnitude and apparent reproducibility of the claimed effects. The need to determine the reproducibility of antecedent results in independent laboratories is essential, regarding the general importance of oxidative stress as a causative factor in many human diseases (Cutler 2005). Thus, we recruited a group of highly experienced and prominent biofield therapy practitioners to participate in a series of experiments, treating cells exposed to H_2O_2. Importantly, the fact that all of the practitioners were inclined to participate in the studies at various institutions paved the way for future attempts to replicate the experiments reported here.

The standardization of the independent parameters (biofield projections) in bioenergetic interventions is very hard and complex and in the precise form, impossible. Biofield is a combination of various waves with various frequencies and intensities which fluctuate moment to moment because of changing the situational, chronobiological, emotional, cognitive, spiritual, and intentional states. However, the biofield is not a vibrational remedy with a constant formulation. This complexity and uncertainty does not arise from the limitations of methods and instruments of measurement, but because of the chaotic nature of the biofield.

On the other hand, several studies indicate that biofield projection can be controlled and that there are reliable and valid congruence between intention and psychophysical effects. Regulation of frequency and intensity of biofield is performed in an intra/inter/transpersonal context and organized qualitatively (not quantitative).

How the intentional bioenergy interventions are generated, projected, and transferred to their related psychophysical pathways and produce the specific effects, still remains an enigma. Some of the bioenergy-based therapies exert their specific effects via stimulation of special physical gates of energetic body like acupoints in acupuncture and acupressure or chakras stimulation in yoga and Qigong, and/or some of them control the specific effects via controlling or selecting the vibrational factors like homeopathy (selected vibrational medicines) or acupressure (controlling the manner of manipulation) and all of the hands-on, hands-off, and distant interventions which are performed by controlling the thought field.

Another controversial problem is that on the condition that environmental fields can exert no biological effects unless the energy intensity is sufficient to ionize or heat tissues (Foster & Pickard 1987; Wachtel 1995), how can weaker fields, such as human biofield, effect significant and specific biological changes?

From Qidynamic viewpoint, a physics/biology dilemma is propounded in this problem.

Oschman (2000b) pointed out that this physics/biology dilemma was resolved when careful research revealed that biological systems completely defy a simple and obvious logic: "Larger stimuli should produce large responses." In living systems, extremely weak fields have potent effects, while there may be little or no response to strong fields. A turning point in the controversy came about when scientists from the prestigious Neurosciences Research Program examined the evidence and concluded:

A striking range of biological interactions has been described in experiments where control procedures appear to have been adequately considered. The existence of biological effects of very weak electromagnetic fields suggests an extraordinarily efficient mechanism for detecting these fields and discriminating them from much higher levels of noise. The underlying mechanisms must necessarily involve ever-increasing number of elements in the sensing system, ordered in particular ways to form a cooperative organization and to manifest similar forms and levels of energy over long distances (Adey & Bawin 1977).

This statement marked the emergence of a new paradigm in biology that has led to extensive research and clinical investigations into the beneficial and harmful effects of electromagnetic fields. We now know that cells and tissues are highly nonlinear, non-balanced, cooperative and coherent systems, capable of responding to very specific "windows" in terms of frequency and intensity (Adey 1990).

Figure 4.2 shows Qidynamic windows which determine selective responses of the brain to electromagnetic pulses.

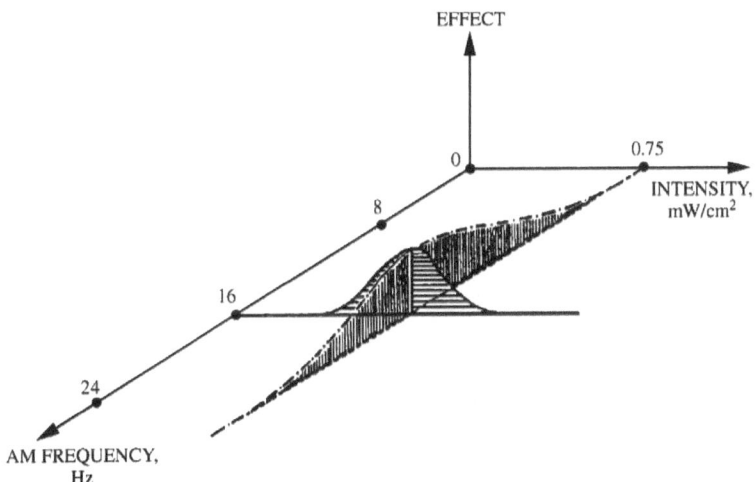

Figure 4.2. A frequency-power window. The frequency-power-density "window" or "response surface" for the brain. The measured response was calcium-ion efflux from forebrain tissue. The fundamental signal frequency was 147 MHz (million cycles per second). This signal was amplitude modulated sinusoidally at selected frequencies and power densities. This study, published by Blackman and colleagues (1979), confirmed earlier work by Bawin and colleagues (1975) who reported that brain tissue has maximum frequency

sensitivity in the ELF range, between 6 and 20 Hz and intensity of 10^{-7} V/crn. This is the level associated with navigation and prey detection in marine vertebrates and with control of human biological rhythms. The amplitude modulated microwave signal has an intensity window around 10^{-7} V/crn. This is at the level of the electroencephalogram (EEG) in brain tissue. Also see Adey (1980). The illustration is redrawn from Blackman CF, Elder JA, Weil CM, Benane SG, Eichinger DC, and House DE 1979 Induction of calcium-ion efflux from brain tissue by radio-frequency radiation: Effects of modulation frequency and field strength. Radio Science 14: 93-98 (quoted from Oschman 2000b, With kind permission from AGU).

Biomedical researchers have been testing the use of pulsing magnetic fields originating outside the organism to induce microcurrents within tissues to enhance healing. A consistent observation is that triggering a cellular response requires the application of energy in a very narrow range of frequencies and intensities (Bassett 1978 and 1995).

Bioelectromagnetics has shown that organisms including microbes may respond to externally applied, extremely weak electromagnetic fields and even those of less-energy content than the physical thermal noise limit (Rubik et al. 1994; Rubik, Brooks & Schwartz 2006).

Gradually, the evidence confirming that the biophysical mechanisms involved in the amplification of tiny signals produce significant physiological and behavioral effects accrued cumulatively (Ho & Knight 1998; Ho, Popp & Warnke 1994).

Field effects are highly specific and confined to a narrow power-frequency window. Oschman (1998) noted the similarity between the frequencies and intensities of low-energy emissions from the hands of therapists, on the one hand, and the signals from pulsed electromagnetic field (PEMF) devices used in clinical medicine, on the other hand. Medical researchers have documented a cascade of signal transduction processes from the cell membrane to the nucleus and onto the genetic material that are facilitated by PEMF therapies (Bassett 1995). Polarity touch, Reiki, therapeutic touch, acupuncture, and many hands-on/off therapies probably affect the same signal pathways.

These findings corroborate the biological effects of subtle vibrational interventions and remind us of an ancient Taoistic dictum: "The finest is the most powerful."

Nonlinear and highly selective responses of biological parameters to biofields and environmental fields shift our mind from a mechanical paradigm to a cyber semiotic paradigm. Each signal is interpreted in a differential organization (various windows), and if it produces a meaningful stimulation, a specific psychophysical pathway will be activated.

Although various signals are utilized in medicine, most of the studies are focused on extremely low frequency (ELF, less than 100 Hz) and low-energy electromagnetic fields (Miller 1986). The frequencies which are recorded from Qi emissions of healer's hands are in ELF range (Oschman 2000a; Wu 1997).

Of course, the human biofield contains different frequencies, each with its specific effects on biological parameters.

ELF frequencies, dependent on their range, fasciitate healing of different types of tissues. Figure 4.3 illustrates a signal recorded by John Zimmerman from the hand of a practitioner of therapeutic touch (Zimmerman 1990). The signal frequency was not steady, but varied from 0.3 to 30 Hz, with most of the activity in the range of 7-8 Hz. Figure 4.3 also shows the portions of the "sweep" that correspond to some of the clinical results (Oschman 2000a).

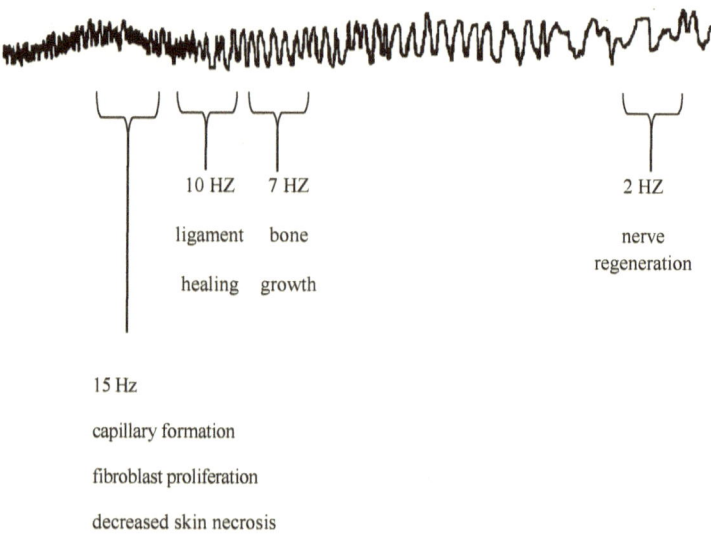

Figure 4.3. Signal recorded by Dr. John Zimmerman from the hand of a practitioner of therapeutic touch. The frequency was not steady, but varied from 0.3 to 30 Hz, with most of the activity in the range of 7-8 Hz. The second wide brackets show portions of the "sweep" that approximately correspond to some of the clinical results (quoted from Oschman 2000a, With permission of Elsevire).

But infrared waves, which are emitted from Qigong healers, enhance the growth of cells, protein production, and cellular ventilation (Mackean 1973). There are evidences which indicate living matter can generate microwaves (Enander & Larson 1977) and light (Oschman 1998; Rattemeyer, Popp & Nagl 1981).

Cellular Qidynamics

Most of the Qidynamic effects can be explained via modulating intracellular free calcium as a ubiquitous second messenger in various physiological systems.

Several studies concentrate on the direct effects of biofields on CNS (Anderson & Anderson 1968; Oschman 2000a; Wisneski 1997) or ANS (Mackay, Hansen & McFarlane 2004), but the living matrix network seems to be more appropriate and widespread bioenergy transduction (see e.g., Frohlich 1988; Ho & Knight 1998; Ingber 1993).

However, the dynamics of biofield through the living matrix or nervous system can be mediated by Na^+/Ca^{2+} exchanger and calcium meridian (Kiang, Ives & Jonas 2005). Some of the studies focus on calcium ions changing in thalamocortical neurons as electromagnetic pacemaker (Destexhe, Babloyantz & Sejnowski 1993; Wallenstein 1994) and some other focus on pineal as the external/inducer master gland (Wisneski 1997).

Biofield can increase intracellular free calcium all over the body via the living matrix signaling. Ca^{2+} is an important transuding signal in the cell, which increases in resting intracellular free calcium concentration ($[Ca^{2+}]_i$) and triggers a variety of cell functions including metabolism, growth, differentiation, hormonal secretion, gene expression, protein synthesis, and cell movement (Kiang & Tsokos 1998; Meldolesi & Pozzan 1987). It is known that $[Ca^{2+}]_i$ is maintained by three main mechanisms: the influx of extracellular Ca^{2+}, Ca^{2+}-binding proteins in the cytoplasm, such as calmodulin, and Ca^{2+} release from intracellular pools, such as the endoplasmic reticulum, mitochondria, and Golgi apparatus. The endoplasmic reticulum comprises inositol 1, 4, 5-trisphosphate that is generated by a membrane transduction process including a receptor, a coupling G protein, and phospholipase C, whereas influx of extracellular Ca^{2+} is through voltage-gated, second messenger-mediated, or receptor-mediated Ca^{2+} meridians (Berridge & Irvine 1989).

The EBE-induced increase in $[Ca^{2+}]_i$ is also mediated by L-type voltage-gated Ca^{2+} meridian because both external K^+ at a high concentration and the L-type voltage-gated Ca^{2+} meridian blocker verapamil significantly increased the basal $[Ca^{2+}]_i$ and abolished the EBE-induced increase in $[Ca^{2+}]_i$. This observation is unique to the EBE effects because exposure of cells to heat stress (Kiang, Koenig & Smallridge 1992) or NaCN (Kiang & Smallridge 1994) activates only the Na^+/Ca^{2+} exchanger. Activation of L-type voltage-gated Ca^{2+} has been shown in dorsal root ganglion—neuroblastoma hybrid ND8-47 cells (Tang, Kiang & Cox 1994). It is possible that Jurkat T cells possess properties of both systemic cells and neuronal cells.

The EBE-induced increase was also blocked by verapamil, an L-type voltage-gated Ca^{2+} meridian blocker. These results suggest that the EBE-induced $[Ca^{2+}]_i$ increase may serve as an objective means for assessing and validating bioenergy effects and dignifying those specialists who have a claim to bioenergy capability (Kiang et al. 2002). The increase in $[Ca^{2+}]_i$ is mediated by activation of Na^+/Ca^{2+} exchangers and opening of L-type voltage-gated Ca^{2+} meridians.

Nonlocal Dynamics

It seems that expert healers and skillful self-healers can modify the biofield modalities intentionally via stimulation of specific energy centers and points and/or by psycho-biofeedback mechanisms, which generates and amplifies proper frequencies and intensities in order to activate specific psychoneuroimmunological pathways. Intentionality, if administered directly and via the cognitive and behavioral modifications, can switch the specific frequency-power windows to induce ideal psychophysical changes.

A range of the so-called target systems has been used to study the possible effect of distant intentionality on living systems, with a range of possible studies that is nearly as diverse as the processes within an organism that might be influenced. Research participants have included healers, psychics, and unselected laboratory volunteers. The existing literature shows the typical stages of a research paradigm, moving from less to more systematic research over a period of forty years. Despite vast differences in the database of more than 150 studies, the experiments generally fall into two major categories (Schlitz & Braud 1997).

The first category is a direct analog of actual healing practices. It consists of studies in which a healer seeks to influence and mitigate a deleterious process or condition in a target organism. The aim is to improve the organism's vitality or decrease its morbidity. For example, biologist Bernard Grad, a pioneer in this field of study, watered seeds with saline solution that had been treated by a healer or solution that had not. In a careful, double-blind design, Grad found that the seeds watered with healer-treated saline were more likely to sprout and grow successfully.

Another biologist, Carroll Nash, reported that the growth rate of bacteria could be influenced by conscious intention in controlled, double-blind studies. Likewise, psychological researcher William Braud found a highly significant reduction, attributable to the effect of intention, in hemolysis rates of the participant's own blood cells held in a saline solution in test tubes in a distant room.

Some studies in this category involved an attempt to influence the course of a naturally occurring disease or condition. For instance, healers have successfully reduced the growth of cancerous tumors in laboratory animals, compared with growth rates of unhealed control animals. In another example, volunteers successfully minimized complications related to heart disease in hospitalized patients, compared with untreated control patients. It is in this latter case that we find a research that bears the closest resemblance to healing per se (Schlitz & Braud 1997).

A second major category of distant intentionality on living systems involves the measurement of ongoing normal processes or behaviors in target organisms. The typical experiments are designed to have either neutral or beneficial effects. The research includes effects on long-term factors such as growth of plants or cell cultures and short-term changes in motor behavior or physiological activity. For practical reasons, the study of ongoing normal processes has received the most experimental attention.

In particular, numerous studies have addressed the question of whether physiological measures—specifically autonomic nervous system activity in humans—might be susceptible to distant intentionality. In one series of experiments, electrodermal activity (EDA) fluctuations were chosen as the physiological measure. Such measurements are readily made sensitive indicators which are known to be useful peripheral measures of the activity of the measures represent a coherent and methodologically consistent subset of the overall database of studies of the influence of distant intentionality on living systems (ibid).

The pure intentional interventions as appear in distance healing have been established via several valuable studies, but dynamisms and mechanisms of these phenomena have been unknown.

Some theories as quantum nonlocality and Bohm's implicate order explain synchronized and nonlocal interactions which are observed in prayer and other types of distance healing (Bohm 1980; Rohrlich 1983). The quantum fluctuations of virtual and real particles give rise to interference patterns that specifically link separated submicroscopic particles, and this, in turn, implies a functional interconnection on larger scales (Ibison & Haisch 1996; Preparata 1995). A consequence of this quantum inseparability is that physical systems exhibit a quality of wholeness, as suggested in Bohm's work (Bohm 1980). While not explanatory in a mechanistic sense, such models bring consciousness into the picture with an efficacious role. They suggest that we, as observers, are a necessary ingredient in the determination of physical reality.

Extensions of this modeling approach consider more directly the informational theoretical aspects of anomalous interactions. In a version of quantum theory that emphasizes the interconnection and wholeness of the physical world, Bohm describes a particular form of "active" information that is potentially present everywhere, but which is active only where it is meaningful (Bohm 1980). Thus, a healing intent may be available as an information resource which owns a nonlocal, and universal extension, in conjunction with the need for healing foster the meaning, and hence the resonant meridian, through which the information becomes active.

Taking consciousness as a form or manifestation of information, Jahn and Dunne advance a metaphoric extension of quantum mechanical principles into the consciousness domain (Dunne & Jahn 1987; Jahn & Dunne 1986). Consciousness is regarded as both particulate and wavelike, in analogy with quantum mechanical descriptions of matter and energy. In its nonlocallized, wavelike manifestation, it is unbounded and can penetrate barriers and resonate with other consciousnesses and the environment, thereby acquiring or inserting information that is unique to the interacting system (Nelson 1999).

Several models try to describe the local and nonlocal effects of consciousness and how intentions change the matter via behaviors or without any objective media. M^5 model (modular model of mind/matter manifestations) is one of these theoretical frameworks which is simply explicative of normal an anomalous mind—matter pathways (Jahn 2001).

The essence of the M^5 model is sketched in figure 4.4, which illustrates four conceptual modules juxtaposed in a rectangular array, wherein:

Ⓒ Denotes all pertinent functions of the conscious mind of the operator, including perception, representation, cognition, memory, volition, activation, etc., as usually treated in the cademic formulations of psychology, neurophysiology, and philosophy.

(T) Encompasses all of the events and processes of the tangible physical world, as commonly represented in the natural sciences and the technological and medical applications thereof.

(U) Subsumes all mental processings commonly termed "unconscious," "subconscious," or "preconscious," including both procedural aspects, such as storage of information and experiences, autonomic control of physiological functions, subliminal reactions to stimuli, instinctive behavior and insight, and preparation for conscious attention and action, as well as "dynamic" aspects, such as protection from trauma and other experiential overloads.

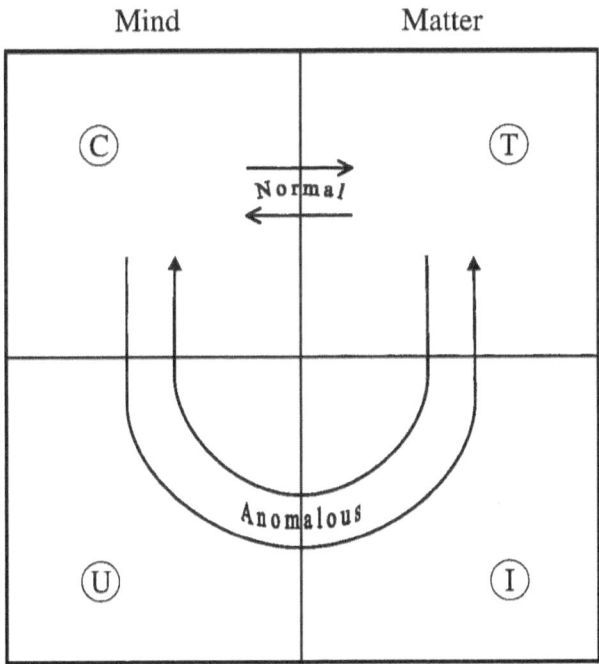

Figure 4.4. Modular model of mind/matter manifestations (quoted from Jahn, 2001, With kind permission from Dr. Jahn)

(I) Refers to an intangible or subtangible level of physical events and processes purported to underlie the tangible or observable phenomena of the natural world. This domain has been conceptualized, labeled, and analyzed in various abstruse theoretical frameworks, e.g., "quantum holism," "implicate order," "ontic level," "string theory," "vacuum or ZPF physics," etc., all of which share the presumption of a premanifest basis or source for all tangible phenomena, wherein the common parameters of substance, energy, and information; space and time; and even mind and matter are undiscriminated.

The essential proposition of the M^5 model, then, is that rather than exercising "normal" modes of information transfer directly from C to T, or *vice versa*, mind/matter anomalies are achieved by more circuitous routes, wherein consciousness invokes its unconscious capabilities, and tangible events diffuse into their intangible counterparts, allowing the intrinsic indistinguishability of the mental and material aspects at their deepest levels to provide the bridge that completes the information circuit (Jahn 2001).

Qidynamic Analysis of Bioenergy-Based Therapies

Above-mentioned documents and theories lead us to believe a matter-energy-information-consciousness continues flow between various levels of organization locally and nonlocally.

These facts and models are summarized in figure 4.5 as a Qidynamic analysis model which shows various tapes of biofield interventions and several stages of bioenergy-based healing response.

Intentionality resources can be either "autogenic" like different techniques of healing meditation and imagery or "proximal" as therapeutic touch and other hands-on/off therapies, or "distal" such as prayer and various distance healing techniques. Nonlocal biofields affect the organism through the implicate order; the domain of quantum holism wherein actions and events can be synchronized and coordinated with each other in a nonlocal manner.

The vectors show the mutual intra/inter/transpersonal matter-energy-information-consciousness interactions which induce healing response in the afferent pathway and modulate the energy-information gateways and pathways and finally affect the intentionality resources.

Some of the bioenergy healing systems employ only one kind of intentional biofield intervention like prayer (distal) or therapeutic touch (proximal) but other systems such as Reiki, Qigong of yoga administer more than one resource.

Establishing the bioenergetic economy entails an interdisciplinary method, (physics, medicine, psychology, and ontology) to employ all of the healing resources in an integrative clinical setting and without any superfluous assumptions.

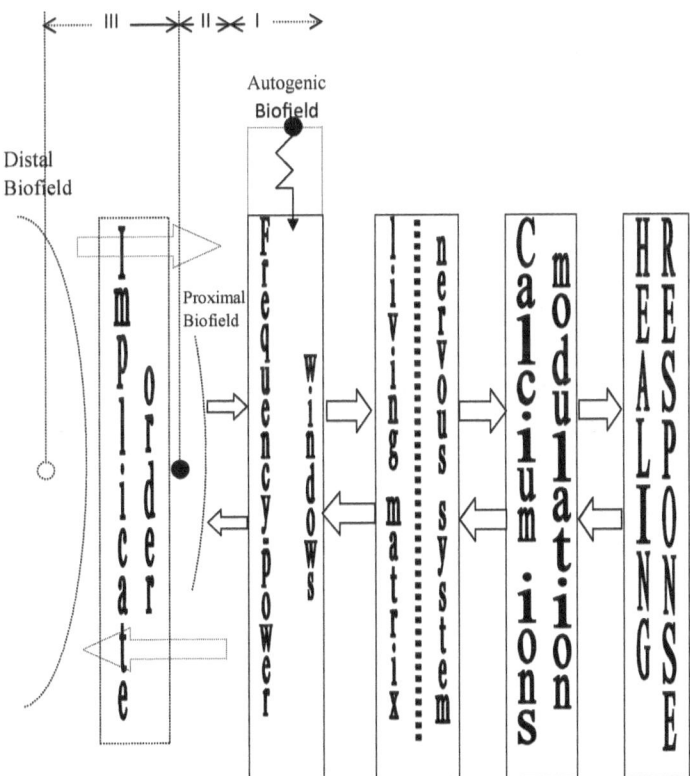

Figure 4.5. A simplified Qidynamic analysis model of various types of intentional biofield interventions

The mutual vectors show the intra/inter/transpersonal matter-energy-information-consciousness interactions. I=Intrapersonal space, II=Interpersonal space, III=Transpersonal space.

Qikinetics

Healing response to Qidynamic procedure is a biopsychosociospiritual response, which is considered in Qikinetics.

Qikinetics studies the alternations of Qidynamic effects in an intra/inter/transpersonal context and also explains the effects of nonbioenergetic components of bioenergy-based therapies which interface with bioenergy-induced dynamisms. Some of the researchers may deem the Qikinetic phenomena as nonspecific effects of biofield healings. Nonetheless, it must be heeded that each of the bioenergy healing systems in addition to intentional bioenergy interventions contains physical, ethical, spiritual, philosophical, and psychological components. As a result of the complexity of these interventional matrices, there is no systematic and analytical study on effectiveness of each component of these systems.

In the discussion, which ensues, we describe only the common aspects of bioenergy healing systems from a methodological viewpoint. Some of them are considered as specific effects of general qualitative and communicative components of biofield healing. Believe in mind-body, man—nature, and illness/healing-life unity and so emphasizing on healing presence and inner healing power are basic assumptions and inductions of these systems which can evoke healing response intra/inter/transpersonally.

Concerning these aspects, efficacy of energetic approaches can be expounded on the basis of the following biopsychosocial pathways:

Intra/interpersonal mechanisms:

1.1. Classic conditioning
1.1.1. Placebo effect
1.1.2. Indirect suggestions
1.2. Operant conditioning
1.3. Abstract conditioning
1.4. Immune conditioning (PNI)

1.5. Beliefs system
1.6. Relaxation response

Transpersonal mechanisms:

2.1. Communicative biofields
2.2. Presence experiences

Although these fields may have imbrications with each other, this classification can be of use to analyze therapeutic elements of energetic approaches. In the following, each of the above-mentioned dynamics will be explained briefly:

As it was mentioned, these therapeutic processes are absolutely dependent on the individual and can be activated with or without the intervention of external factors. Nonetheless, as awareness, skill, and self-effectiveness are not usually sufficient, the individual is not able to control these intrinsic healing mechanisms. As a result, this ability is projected to a special person or situation that is believable for the individual to be the cause of these processes.

1. Intra/Interpersonal Mechanisms
1.1. Classical Conditioning

When a neutral stimulus is frequently accompanied by stimulus (unconditional stimulus), that naturally elicits a response (unconditional response) until the neutral stimulus (conditional stimulus) can solely elicit the response (conditional response), classical conditioning happens.

This mechanism can be activated either via providing therapeutic factors and presenting the content of a therapeutic approach or as a result of context factors such as the physical and symbolic atmosphere.

In the following, the conditioning and content effects as well as the placebo, context conditioning, or indirect suggestion effects are briefly explained.

1.1.1. Placebo Effect

The term "placebo" was first used by Osler in nineteenth century (Rodgers 2001). Placebo is defined as any therapeutic agent that is administered to have therapeutic effects on a symptom or disease, but in fact it is inert or has a nonspecific effect on that symptom or disease (Shapiro & Shapiro 1997).

Placebo effects and their cognitive mediating mechanisms, especially with regard to the healee and others in the surrounding caring environment in the context of healing presence, requires a more punctilious inspection (Caspi & Bootzin 2002). Expectancy is contextual, individual, dyadic, or intimately systemic and sociocultural (Walach et al. 2002) and is likely governed by experience and relevancy within these levels of interaction (So 2002). Expectancies have variable impact upon health outcomes that in some contexts may be significant (Kirsch & Sapirstein 1998; Walach 2001). Contemporary research on response shifts indicates that placebo responders may change their perceptions or internal anchors/definitions of health. In response shifts over time, the person's internalized standards for evaluating the same symptom or condition and/or the conceptualization of a target construct such as overall health may alter (Golembiewski, Billingsley & Yeager 1976; Sprangers et al. 1999).

It is believed by some that placebo effect is effective only on imaginative symptoms such as pain, but Esgate and Groome (2001) in various studies have demonstrated that objective parameters such as the results of blood tests, infectious and inflammatory diseases, wound healing, and body temperature are influenced by placebo.

Although the placebo effect has been known for many years and has been applied extensively in many case-control studies, it has been studied and used appropriately (Harrington 1997).

In the research in interventions that impact the whole organism and activate the organism's regulatory and self-healing capacities, expectancy may play a particularly more prominent role alteration of context. For example, double-blind versus naturalistic or outcome-based research models may alter expectancy (Walach 2001). Patient expectations play a central role in behavioral and psychoneuroimmunological changes as the main initiator and supportive parameter of placebo effects (figure 4.6).

Actually, in placebo effect the effective factor in healing is a symbolic element that all of its effects cannot be mentioned nonspecific as it can specifically stimulate neuropsychoimmunology system. A factitious method or a sham surgery is effective with just the same mechanism.

This symbolic element is present in all effective agents or interventions, and all treatments lend a significant portion of its effect to placebo effect. In our classification, that part of effective factors that are directly presented as therapeutic intervention is brought under the entity of placebo effect.

In energetic treatments, the attendance of the therapist, displaying illumination, and believing that the patient is now under the effect of a healing energy field can have placebo effect even if the transfer does not happen or the therapist is not expert or his energy field is not at the therapeutic range of inducing effect (much less than 7-8 Hz). Even in such cases patients have reported some degrees of recovery.

The historical and cultural backgrounds that lend credence to it enhance the passive state that occurs automatically during the process of energy reception as well as the individual's suggestibility. Moreover, reports of recovery of other patients greatly augment the placebo effect of energetic approaches.

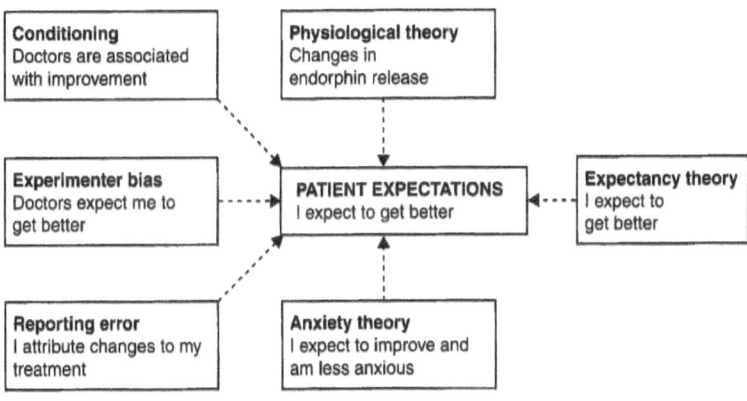

The central role of patient expectations in placebo effects

Figure 4.6. The central role of patient expectations in placebo effects (quoted from Ogden 2004, With kind permission from Dr. Ogden)

1.1.2. Indirect Suggestions

Despite the popular notion that hypnosis is a unique psychological state which needs trace and direct suggestions, all of us have frequently experienced hypnosis naturally and without any direct suggestion.

Modern clinical hypnosis is more often carried out via indirect, metaphoric suggestion in no trance hypnotherapy as different studies have proved that these methods causes less resistance and more permanent effects (Gordon 1978; Hammond 1990).

Each therapeutic method has its special indirect implications and metaphors, and in this way, the physical and symbolic context and atmosphere in which the therapeutic intervention takes place can be specified to mind-body dynamics.

In energetic treatments, the following metaphors are transferred to the individual in an implicit manner during the familiarity course, treatment and follow-up, all of which can induce mental and physical effects:

a) Individual-therapist-universe energetic linkage.
b) Fluidity of the energetic body instead of rigidity of physical body.
c) Healing as a natural characteristic of human organism.
d) Healing process as an organic process not dependent to the therapeutic factor.
e) Healing current as a ubiquitous current in universe.

These therapeutic metaphors, regardless of their theoretical, philosophical, and practical importance which were explained before, are so effective and leads the individual from an alienation state to a feeling of safety resulting from the link with universe and others [suggestions (a) and (e)]. Hence, the concern for inability to change the future would be resolved and the patient will trust his organism in treatment and commit the natural process of evolution and healing (c and d). Thus, instead of considering physical injuries which are irreversible as a result of rigid attitude toward the body, concerns the disorder as a fluid energetic disorder that can be recovered by changing its health pattern (b).

These suggestions can enhance the stability of autonomous nervous system, activate neuropsychoimmunology system appropriately and control the health behaviors in favor of health.

1.2. Operant Conditioning

A psychophysical feedback is the basic mechanism for adjusting the bioenergy healing techniques to with the healing intentions and individual differences. On the other hand, positive reinforcement of healing intention and healing response emanates from positive feedbacks of the other healees.

Group therapy sessions and self-help groups are very common in the bioenergy-based therapies and presentation of healing case reports and personal experiences enhanced the healing response in participants.

1.3. Abstract Conditioning

The definition of abstract conditioning was experimentally presented by Corn-Becker, Welch, and Fisischelli (1949).

This type of conditioning is mainly used to explain the mechanism of hypnosis (Crasilneck & Hall 1985). The validity of what are expressed during this type of conditioning is proved by consequent experiments. In other words, abstract conditioning is acceptance of the statement before testing it. Thus, the individual believes in the antecedent, and so it is assimilated to his mind and established there; this belief makes the antecedent to be realized in an objective and psychomotoric way. Consequently, the outcome of this induction is objectively accomplished through psycho-physical mechanisms.

During the process of receiving bioenergy, most people experience different sensations such as heat, burning, or paresthesia or the feeling of a current of magnetic field, which are usually new for them. Patients generally report some degrees of recovery in symptoms or disease after these experiences. The question is as follows: Do these experiences during energy reception indicate a physical or physiological effect? Or the relationship between these experiences and recovery is a symbolic and conditioned link?

The new experience of bioenergy reception can act as a hypnotic suggestion, and receiving energy and being healing can make it believable. As a result, the patient feels some degrees of recovery, and after this according to classical conditioning, the patients consider this experience as recovery, and the response will be facilitated more.

1.4. Immune Conditioning and Psychoneuroimmunology

Another basic science that tries to define the relation of mind-body and understand the unity of human organism is psychoneuroimmunology, which was developed as a result of increase in our objective and quantitative understanding of the linkage of genetic, structural, and functional aspects of nervous system as well as hormonal and immunity systems, the effect of neural and hormonal mediators on immune cells and vice versa, and also the influence of psychologic states on neuronal, hormonal, and immunity performance. Laboratory and clinical studies have revealed the relationship of these systems and completed the puzzle of integrated system of psychoneuroimmunology. By development of this science, medicine seems to be more ready than ever to experience an evolution by linking its clinical and theoretical separate elements. This evolution is in the direction of giving importance to role, relation, patient, and generally the immune modulating in prevention and treatment of diseases (Goli 2003b).

The term *psychoneuroimmunology* was first used by Robert Ader, which was focused on the relation of nervous and immune systems. In the second revision of his book *Psychoneuroimmunology*, he defined this science as follows:

Much scientific evidence confirms that nervous system is linked with immune system from neuroanatomical, neuroendocrine, and neurochemical points of view. The bilateral relation of immune and nervous systems justifies a series of experimental findings in relation with the effect of behavioral stress-dependent changes and conversely the effect of immunological processes on behavior (Ader, Felten & Cohen 1991).

In consequent studies, it has been shown how psychologic stresses can change immunological performance, number of immune cells, and also the amount of secretion of immune mediators as well as the predisposition of individuals to be affected by diseases (Glaser et al. 1997; Rood et al. 1993). On the other hand, mood disorders can impair the immunological performance (Bartlett et al. 1995; Evans et al. 1992; Irwin et al. 1990).

Studies on human model and also human have shown that immune system can be affected by conditioned reflexes, and by conditioning, the performance of immune system can be enhanced or deteriorated. This process is called immune conditioning. This process has been even employed in immune suppression for treatment of cancer (Bovbjerg et al. 1990).

This psychoimmunological finding reveals the mind-body relation from another point of view and provides the basis for further laboratory and clinical research in many immuno-modulation methods. Effectiveness of these methods on immunological performance have been demonstrated by studies on the modulating effects of relaxation techniques (Hall et al. 1996; Hall, Minnes & Olness 1993; Hall et al. 1984), hypnosis on delayed sensitivity reactions (Kiecolt-Glaser et al. 1986), reaction to HSV1 (Locke et al. 1994), and number of natural killer cells (NKC) (Zachariae et al. 1990; 2005).

These studies imply that the relation of mind and body factors in cognitive and behavioral aspects of physical diseases is a robust and provable hypothesis. This relationship is emphasized in complementary and alternative medicine methods and considered weak and unimportant in biomedicine.

These finding makes the analysis of some of the mechanisms of energetic approaches to health possible. Although bioenergy-based therapies are based on deep and effective relation and paying attention to transpersonal events, such relation can cause deep psychological effect and subsequently immunological results. On the other hand, practical experiments of bioenergy flow and its transfer from the therapist can cause immunity modulation and, as a result, healing of the individual, just the same as inductive and hypnotic effects. The direct effect of induced energy on cells and especially nervous system cannot improve the mood and reduce anxiety. These changes in psychological system on the basis of the above-mentioned mechanisms can treat physical diseases.

The three above-mentioned mind-body mechanisms—effects of cognitive and behavior factors, inductive factors, and bioenergetic—can modulate and control the immune system (Goli 2008).

Concerning the importance of psychoneuroimmunological events is predisposing the individual to diseases, the basic hypothesis of traditional medicine of defining disease and health on the basis of "dynamic balance of internal environment" again become important, and the role of environmental factors fades. From this point of view, it can be said that health is the psychoneuroimmunological equilibrium (ibid).

1.5. Belief System

As physical, human, and symbolic atmosphere are considered the background and context of effectiveness of placebo effect, the belief system is a larger background which direct and indirect suggestions act in and via that.

Our intelligence, health, relations, creativity, happiness, and personal status can be formed, influenced, or even determined by belief. The effective beliefs in health can be categorized into the three groups of beliefs related to reason, meaning, and identity (Dilts, Hallbom & Smith 1991).

Two patients in which one of them believes that the etiology of his disease, genetic, microbes, or any other cause, which is not in his control and the other one who believes that his disease is a result of his lifestyle or impairment of energy balance, would have two completely different behavior and mood system. The first patient will have impulsive behaviors with irregular pattern regarding the feeling of not having control, while the second one will have a more active role, higher inspiration, and consequently may be higher life expectancy. Will the patient who considers his disease as a result of unluckiness or as a messenger of exhaustion and destruction have the same disease-oriented behaviors and psychoneuroimmunological responses with the one who regards the disease as a chance for growth and personality and cognitive evolution? Moreover, will the person who regards himself separated from the universe have the same physiological behaviors and reactions with the one who concerns himself as a part of the universe?

Contemplating over the effect of these beliefs on psychoneuro-immunological responses show that the biomedicine pattern includes many disease causing suggestions. On the other hand, it demonstrates that a significant portion of the effectiveness of holistic interventions such as energetic approaches come from their health-oriented belief system. Many scientists have analyzed the placebo effect in the framework of belief system. Diagram 4.6 explore the placebo effect pathways and also summarizes different viewpoints about the effects of suggestion and belief effects on health (Ogden 2004).

Spirituality is the main belief of the bioenergy-based therapies. Spirituality, belief in a power apart from one's own existence, implies a connection with a universal force transcending every day sense-bound reality. Spirituality defines the search for purpose and meaning (Connor, Davidson & Lee 2003). The impact of the healer's spiritual beliefs on healing presence and on the healee's experience of healing, as well as the interaction of the spiritual beliefs of the healer and healee, are areas of investigation that have received scant attention in the literature. Does a healer's spirituality impact their capacity to be a "healing presence"? In Native American (Suarez, Raffaelli & O'Leary 1996) and ancient cultures and practices [Cameron 2001; Dhonden 2000), and Ayurveda, (Caldecott 2006)], it is common for those who are physically ill to seek spiritual healing from an identified practitioner, the spiritual sage identified as a healer. Contemporary healing therapeutic disciplines (Hover-Kramer 1989; 1996; Johari 1987; Schlitz & Braud 1985) have as foundation the belief in healing by a supernatural force or God and his/her efficacy as healer (Montgomery 1996).

Considering this, the beliefs of an individual about himself, the reason, and meaning of his status as well as his expectations of the treatment process, and so the belief system of health providers makes a symbolic matrix that can develop subjective and objective changes.

1.6. Relaxation Response

In all energetic approaches, the reception status and passive concentration that are the main characteristics of relaxation are suggested directly or indirectly. The relaxation response either causes as a result of formal or informal methods. It will arouse the following behavioral and psychological effects (Benson 1976; Murphy, Donovan & Taylor 1997):

- Enhancement of stress coping ability
- Increasing empathy
- Increasing of self-motivation and independence
- Self-control augmentation
- Perception improvement
- Improvement of concentration
- Development of spirituality

As a result, the response can treat many physical and psychologic disorders such as depression, anxiety, sleep disorders, GI disorders, allergies, cardiovascular diseases, chronic pains, and substance abuse (Astin 1997; Astin 1998; Castillo-Richmond et al. 2000; Edwards 1991; Kabat-Zinn et al. 1998; Zamarra et al. 1996).

It seems that many effects of energetic approaches are dependent on the general relaxation response and the contextual effect of this mind-body status. This contextual effect is so important in the techniques which directly employ direct suggested relaxation and physical, breathing and imaginary exercises as well as the methods in which the patient is in a receptive and passive state; such as healing techniques

2. Transpersonal Mechanisms

Transpersonal psychology is generally regarded as a branch of humanistic psychology, but it seems to have the potential to be considered as an independent approach in psychology.

Carl Gustav Jung was the first who used the term "transpersonal" for collective unconscious phenomena. Grof (1972) defined transpersonal consistent with the viewpoint of Jung:

> "Transpersonal experiment is the experiment which requires extension of conscious beyond the typical boundaries of ego and limitations of time and place."

The consciousness of one can be linked with that of others through which a kind of dialogue and interaction can occur between egos. Passing the ego boundaries provides a kind of integrity between human being and at a higher level between all organisms and the consciousness.

This point is more comprehensible where the importance of therapeutic relation in healing process is understood.

Many therapeutic approaches emphasis on a therapeutic relation accompanied by bilateral trust and respect between the therapist and the patient and believe that without such relation the treatment techniques will not be so effective. A therapist, who does not go beyond the ego and consciousness conventional boundaries, cannot make relation with the emotions and problems of his patient. Such therapist, with a limited view, will only perform symptom therapy and present some medicine and therapeutic techniques and will not move toward the higher values of the patient which is one of the goals of a permanent and effective psychotherapy (see Shamlou 2002).

By believing in such movement in the process of treatment, Maslow (1970) has denoted that transpersonal psychology discusses the higher values and experiences.

Generally, humanistic scientists, by emphasizing the healing nature of transpersonal experiments, link it with the experiences and aspiration that direct people toward transcendence as well as the experiences that relate to their healing potential of self-transcendence (Vaughan 1986).

2.1. Communicative Biofields

As interference of smaller electromagnetic fields of the body form the overall field of the body (Oschman 2000b), interference of fields of different people makes communicative fields by the same mechanism, which is considered as a level of the organization (two person) with its specific function, according to its biopsychosocial view by the same mechanism.

In communication of healer and healee or in group therapies among a group of therapists and patients (some therapists and a patient or a therapist and some patients), an in-phase energetic systems that are open to each other and the universe (higher level of the system) organizes and links the impaired and isolated systems systematically on the basis of the entrainment process.

Different studies have objectively proved the possibility of development of these systems and attunement and entrainment of impaired fields.

Some evidence prove that two persons that sit in a room in front of each other with closed eyes without any physical contact have coordination in their brain and heart rhythm (Beck 1986; Oschman 1993).

In other words, it is possible to dissect reductionistically the elements of healing presence at an interpersonal and intrapsychic level, but the interaction of all of the elements within an intact healer—healee dyad may lead to emergent properties of that dyadic social system (Conveney & Highfield 1995; Gallagher & Appenzeller 1999). Emergent properties are those seen in higher levels of organization but not predicted from the properties of the lower levels of organization (parts) that make up the larger system (Bar-Yam 1997).

Expansion of consciousness to these energetic interactions provides new understanding of the communication as well as ego and ego boundaries.

When the energetic fields of psychotherapist and the client communicate with each other, a meridian to transfer the intuition information is provided. Moreover, the probability of occurrence of deeper therapeutic experiences, which is known as a spiritual experience by the involved individuals, becomes higher (West 2000).

Hall and colleagues (1984), in his explanation of the transfer and reciprocal transfer phenomena, point to the transferring fields both the therapist and client are both influenced by.

Understanding this field is also a deep healing experience, and it seems that regardless of the fact that energy current in its physical definition can affect clients, it can activate the healing process.

Developing coordinated increasing communicative fields, such as energy cycles and attunement experiences, can extend the flow of energy and information beyond the body boundaries effectively. Awareness of these energetic systems provides excellent opportunities in diagnosis and treatment. However, many expert physicians and psychologist take the advantage of these systems without knowing them.

2.2. Presence Experience

In general, two dimensions of presence are described: physical and psychologic, "being there" and "being with" (Gardner 1985). Physical presence involves body-to-body proximity and the requisite skills of seeing, examining, touching, doing, hearing, and hugging or holding. Psychological presence involves mind-to-mind contact (Donough-Means, Kreitzer & Bell 2004).

Carl Rogers, father of humanistic psychology, points to presence experience as an existential in his psychotherapy experiments. About these experiences, he mentioned as follows:

"When I am in changed consciousness status, anything I do is full of healing. Concerning this, my presence is beneficial and saving for clients . . . at this moment, it seems that my inner soul has communicated with the inner soul of the client . . . at these moments, the growth and deep healing energies are present" (Rogers, quoted from Krischenbaum & Henderson 1990).

Rogers's approach was a psychological approach. But as it was mentioned in the integrative health model, when we enter the human organism through any field, other fields will be aroused. The reason for obviousness of Rogers's and other humanistic scientists' energetic experiences was their concern for transpersonal phenomena and the atmosphere between the therapist and client.

Each analysis of presence as an existential, qualitative, and complex experience will be naturally fuzzy, but it is necessary for research and clinical practice.

For this propose, Osterman and Schwartz-Barcott (1996) explicated an appropriate framework to recognize various aspects of presence experience. They explain four levels of presence, which differ in the quality of being there, the focus of energy, the nature of interaction, and positive/negative outcomes. Presence is "being there" in the context of another, physically present, yet not having any level of interaction or involvement. Partial presence is a way of "being there" in which a caregiver is physically located in the context of another and focuses their energy on a task relevant to, but not directly focused on the other. The proliferation of technology in acute care environments may result in caregivers' monitoring machines, minimally interacting with patients, and patients feeling disconnected and isolated interpersonally and interpersonally. Full presence, a way of "being with" in the context of another, includes psychologic as well as physical presence and is the embodiment of empathy, caring, and the use of self in face-to-face interaction. Transcendent presence is the fourth and final level. The exchange of energy between the caregiver and patient is transforming and spiritual in quality and moves beyond the interactional to the transpersonal. Presence is felt as peaceful, comforting, and harmonious, truly more than the therapeutic use of self. Transcendent presence has been achieved when a oneness is felt between caregiver and patient. For purposes of this discussion, transcendent presence may be broadened to include the condition of being physically distant and spiritually present within the quality of being there and healing intention within the focus of energy (Donough-Means, Kreitzer & Bell 2004).

Some of psychologists have mentioned their presence experience as an experience associated with the feeling of unity with the universe, in spite of being separated from it (West 1997; Wilber 1990). However, this separation does not result from alienation, but it is a necessity to develop existential dialogue.

Many psychologists have regarded the Rogers's presence experience so spiritual and beyond reach (West 2000). Nonetheless, in energetic approaches, because of the extension of consciousness of the therapist and the client beyond the boundaries of self or the energy transfer space, the presence experience is so common and achievable.

The bioenergy healing traditions have strong spiritual component, and presence is routinely experienced in both healers and healees. Because of the extensive aspects of the spiritual experiences in bioenergy-based therapies, Wardell and Engebretson (2006) presented a taxonomic analysis on the base of data from a group of healers.

They explicated a structural model of spiritual experience comprised of three domains: circumstances, manifestation, and interpretation. Circumstances included the aspects of setting, situation, and timing. Manifestation incorporated the modes of awareness and the phenomena of the experience. Components of interpretation included personal meaning and congruence with social norms.

Figure 4.7 shows a categorical tree that integrated the data into one framework, reflecting the basic cognitive structure of spiritual experience through which the description of the healers could be presented.

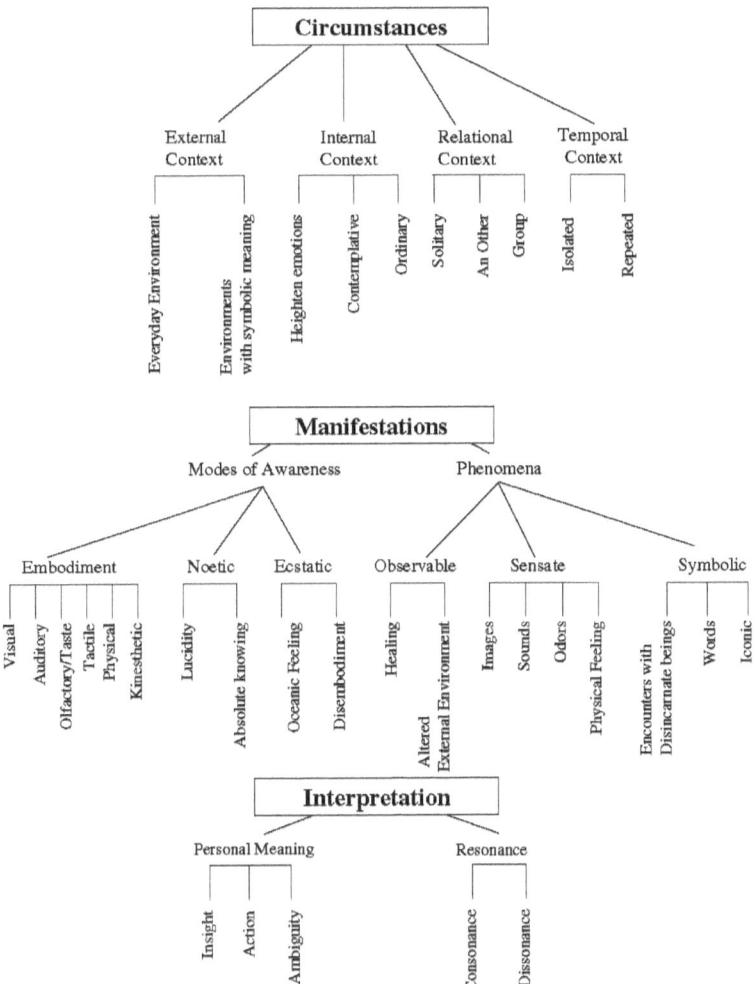

Figure 4.7. Taxonomy of a spiritual experience (quoted from Wardell & Engebretson 2006)

In any case, presence as a spiritual experience provides valuable conditions for healing response, and these analyses, in spite of their defects, help us to design clinical and research programs.

Regarding this, employing energetic approaches in medicine and psychology can help to develop a deep therapeutic relationship and facilitate diagnosis and treatment as well as providing the therapists with significant diagnostic and therapeutic facilities.

Healing and Spectrum of Human Condition

By explaining the intra/inter/transpersonal matrix of healing, we provide an expanded scope of inner healing responses, healer—healee communications, and nonlocal dynamisms. The Qidynamic specific effects and Qikinetic specific/non-specific effects and responses show the expansion of healing response that affect whole person. Several models try to explain this field of effects and responses.

According to McDonough-Means, Kreitzer, and Bell (2004), we need a model to serve as a nidus for heuristic thought in addressing the complex multilevel context of healing response. Figure 4.8 provides a conceptual systemic model to distinct several fields of healing phenomena and is required that integrates knowledge from orthodox fields of research (psychology, sociology, physical and medical sciences, and spirituality) with that which is emerging from biofield medicine research.

Two-dimensional representation of this model is inherently limited in depicting a multidimensional process. The layers in the diagram represent both degree of system complexity (inner to outer or lower to higher) and, in theory, functional relationship with each other. The egg shape or embedding of one within the other reflects the interactive nature of each hierarchy of function and communication. Thus, position should not be viewed as fixed. For example, the bioelectromagnetic layer likely functions with close physical proximity to living beings, could have multiple positions, and just as easily be placed at the next level after physical/chemical level. Similarly, elements of the nonlocal dimension likely impact all less complex layers.

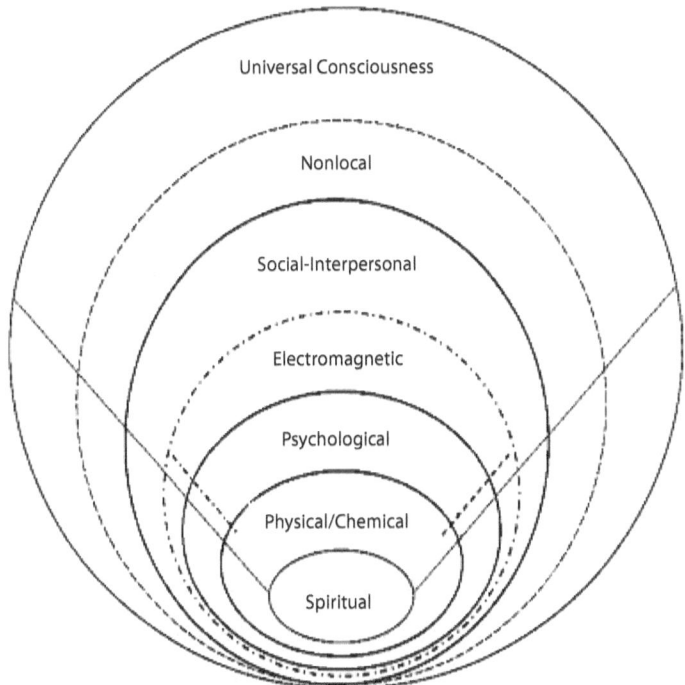

Figure 4.8. Conceptual systemic model. , traditional forces, and lower level of complexity; -----------, nonphysical forces and higher levels of complexity; , likely to be physical forces and regulatory interface; intermediate levels of complexity (quoted from McDonough-Means, Kreitzer & Bell, 2004, With kind permission from Dr. McDonough-Means).

This model describes appropriately the spectrum of the Qidynamics and the Qikinetics effects and responses, but I prefer to adapt and interpret this model to a "phenomenological spectrum of self" from *existential self* as "nothingness experience" to *universal self* as "wholeness experience." The intermediate levels are *physical self*, the matter—energy homeostatic equations, and person as body; *intrapersonal self*, the phenomenal world and person as conscious and unconscious experiences; *etheric self*, the biofield organization and person as vibrational system; *interpersonal self*, the social world and person as behavior, and *transpersonal self*, the world of freewill and person as pure consciousness and implicate order. In spite of the hierarchial shape of this diagram, it is mentionable that nothingness and wholeness are different scopes of the nominal world. The first is experienced in negation way and the other in expansion way of consciousness.

The transpersonal self is the state of man—nature unity where in consciousness is individual and universal simultaneously.

Consciousness is the sum of the "human condition" galaxy, and our conscious mind is the lighted side of the moon which is varied from darkness (unconscious mind) to full moon (conscious mind).

Healer—healee communication is occurred in the intrapersonal self-state and energy-information flow in the self-other relationships (cognitive-behavioral interventions) but healing experience can extend to the communicative biofield and presence experience of the transpersonal level.

Intentions can be evoked from each level but via vibrating the intentional waves all of the levels are affected by degrees. In a biofield healing setting, we focus on conscious intentional biofields. It means that the healing intentions in biofield healing process is originated from conscious mind and extended directly to the vibrational body (local pathway) or indirectly extended to unconscious mind and then affect the vibrational body through the transpersonal level as implicate order (nonlocal pathway) (figure 4.9).

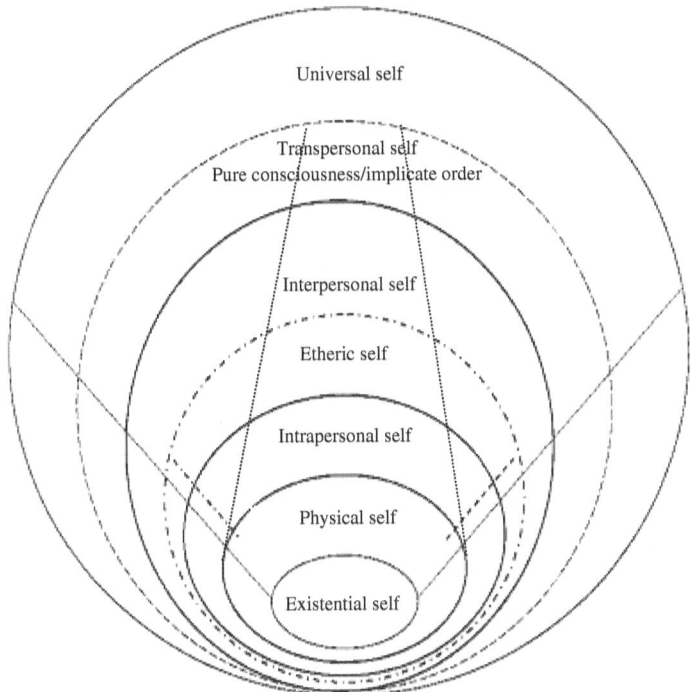

Figure 4.9. The spectrum of human condition; nominal and phenomenal selves.

Biofield healing not only provides a proper clinical setting to modulate the basic level of organization (subatomic) and makes effective changing in health state, but also represents the spectrum of human condition in the clinical practice field. Several aspects of healer—healee communication which were pointed out in this chapter are employed more or less in all forms of therapy but most of the times unconsciously, nonsystematically, and ineffectively.

According to the holistic nature of bioenergetic-based therapies, all of the levels of human condition can be experienced and employed in health promotion.

Chapter **V**

Clinical Basis

Clinical Basis of Energetic Approaches

In holistic approaches to health, a clear border cannot be defined between diagnosis and treatment as well as life and treatment. As it was mentioned before, these approaches are based on enhancement of physical, energetic, psychological, and spiritual balance and also increasing the individual's adaptability with environment. Treatment is considered the secondary result of this process.

In general, energetic approaches are predicated on empathetic relationship with oneself, others—such as patients and the universe. Accordingly, they do not try to diagnose the disease as a primary step in treatment of diseases. According to these approaches, this energetic and spiritual stream will intelligently be absorbed by the points that need it more. Healing streams are directed in a semiconscious, intelligent, or divinely manner, and these servomechanisms do not require our knowledge to guide them.

Pathology of energetic approaches to health is more turn on the pivot of openness and the free activity of Nadis (energy pathways) and chakras (energy centers). However, any abnormality in nutritional habits, social communications, following the moral and spiritual concepts and generally any lifestyle disturbance, can obstruct these pathways and impair the activity of these bioenergy centers. On the other hand, as it was mentioned above, the whole system and not just the impaired center will undergo illumination.

So the pathology of these approaches is not local or disease-oriented as biomedicine.

Treatment is not the goal, but the result of lifestyle modification and the attunement of different biofields with each other, the individual's comprehensive energy field with the therapist, and finally the attunement of biofields with overwhelming energy field and cosmic consciousness.

However, according to the methodology of modern medicine, in this chapter, we will explain some concepts in the three parts of diagnosis, pathogenesis, and treatment to define the clinical aspects of bioenergy healing.

Diagnostic Methods

Since thousands of years ago perspective shamanistic methods were wielded for diagnosis of physical and psychological disorders, but in the history of science, Mathews (1903) has been known as the first one to use energetic fields in diagnosis. He believed that any overactivity in processes or any changes in physical condition of protoplasm of each organ, embryo or zygote, should be construed as an electrical disturbance. These findings have been confirmed by recent studies (Brewitt 1996 and 1999). These studies have demonstrated that not only all normal and pathogenic phenomena make electrical changes in the body, but they also render changes in magnetic fields which surround us. Various studies have evinced that identifying the difference in electromagnetic field and other biofields, which emanate from the obstruction of energy and information pathways in living matrix before any biochemical, histological, and clinical presentation, can identify the etiology of a disease (Brewitt 1996). This can bear witness to the antecedence of energetic changes, as the most basic level of the system, to cellular and molecular changes (Goli 2003a).

Although energetic diagnostic methods, except some few ones such as ECG, EEG, or EMG still have not won approbation in medicine, it seems that diagnosis of energetic disorders can be used as prognostic and economical diagnostic methods.

Besides the objective methods of measurement of biofields, bioenergy practitioners traditionally employ their intuitive methods to diagnose energetic disorders. They believe that they can comprehend the difference between healthy and disturbed biofields, and even their body show some reactions to these disorders (see Astin 1998; Oschman 2000a and 2002).

Regarding this, in the ensuing section, the objective and subjective diagnostic methods in energetic approaches are delineated.

Objective Diagnostic Methods

Objective diagnostic methods are divided to two categories of tools and methods. The quantitative methods record electromagnetic activities of body such as superconduction quantum interference device (SQUID) and more simple magnetometers for recording stronger biofield pulses, which emanate from bioenergy practitioners. On the other hand, the qualitative methods are claimed to image the biofield (aura). These include Kirlian photography, gas discharge visualization (GDV), and polychromatic interference photography (PIP). Now, we will present a brief explanation of the current status of these methods in research and clinical practice.

A—Biofield Recordings

By employing the precise measurement tools of controlling environmental factors and minimizing the human contribution, objective diagnostic methods strive to achieve valid and reliable evaluations.

Over the recent decades, scientists have run the gamut from cynicism to certainty about the presence of energetic fields in the body and surrounding environment. By considering the magnetic fields around body, called biomagnetic fields, biomedicine has utilized diverse equipments.

One of the first equipments of this field traces the magnetic fields of heart (Astin 1998; Oschman 2000a and 2002). This instrument has a coil with two million cycles of wire wound around the axis. This axis is made up of a magnetic material called ferrite. Wires go to an amplifier and recorder.

To obtain quantitative data from electromagnetic fields and body energetic systems, various instruments such as quantum magnetometer and infrared detector are used.

Superconducting quantum interference device (SQUID) includes one or more link of Josephsonian floating in liquid helium. Under appropriate conditions, these connections are extremely sensitive to the environmental magnetic fields. Concerning this, SQUIDs are used in special isolated spaces to avert the intervention of biofields with magnetic fields of environment and the earth (ibid).

SQUIDs and their matrices have found many applications in medical research laboratories to map the biomagnetic fields resulting from the physiological processes inside human body. Moreover, a worldwide network of SQUIDs records the fluctuations of geomagnetic filed every single moment. By using the matrices of SQUID, one can develop three-dimensional images of the energetic field around the body.

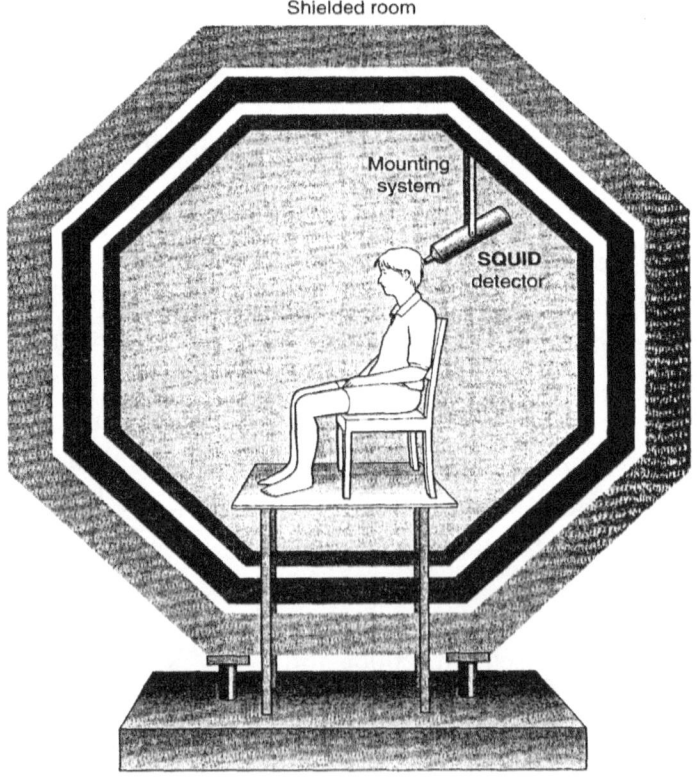

Figure 5.1. Superconducting quantum interference device (SQUID) (from Oschman 2000a, adapted from Takenaka Web site: http//www.takenaka.co.ip/takenaka_e/techno/19_sldrm/19_sldrm.htm, With permission from Elsevire)

Zimmermann and colleagues (1970), by using SQUID, besides completing and developing this instrument, have conducted valuable researches. These studies have constituted a strong connection between the ancient imaginations about energy therapy and modern medicine.

Zimmermann (1990) and Seto and colleagues (1992) also recorded very stronger biomagnetic activities which were only produced by bioenergy healers.

This range of intentional biofield comprises extraordinarily large biomagnetic pulses that emanates from the hands of practitioners of a variety of healing and martial arts techniques in Japan, including Qigong, yoga, meditation, and zen.

The fields were measured with a simple magnetometer consisting of two 80,000 turn coils and a sensitive amplifier. The fields had strength of about 10-3 gauss, which is about one thousand times stronger than the strongest human biomagnetic fields (from the heart), which are about 10-6 gauss and about one lakh times stronger than the fields produced by the brain. Figure 6.5 summarizes the Seto experiment and illustrates a typical recording. As in Zimmerman's study, the biomagnetic field pulsed with a variable frequency centered around 8-10 Hz (Oschman 2000b and 2002).

The work of Zimmerman and Seto has profound implications in terms of correlating ancient concepts of energy medicine with modern science. Neither studies documented any clinical healing during the projection of energy, so further investigation is definitely required. However, the evidence shows that practitioners can emit powerful pulsating biomagnetic fields in the same frequency range that biomedical researchers have determined for jump-starting healing of soft and hard tissue injuries (ibid).

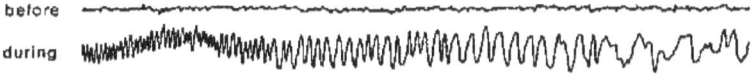

before

during

Figure 5.2. Biomagnetic recording made before and during a therapeutic touch session. During the "healing state," the signal pulsed at a variable frequency, ranging from 0.3 to 30 Hz, with most of the activity in the range 7-8 Hz (quoted from Zimmerman, 1990).

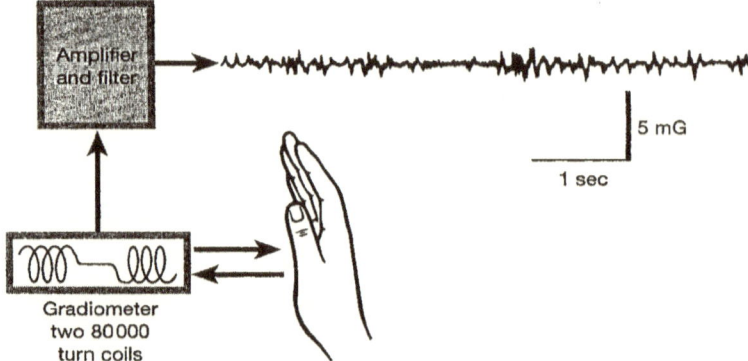

Figure 5.3. Biomagnetic field measurement during "Qi emission" form the hand of a female subject in Tokyo. The double-coil magnetometer recorded a pulsating magnetic field that averaged 2 m gauss, peak to peak, with frequency of 8-10 Hz (quoted from Seto et al, 1992).

B—Biofield Images

A range of devices and techniques are claimed to directly discern and assimilate and to image the aura as the biofield. These include Kirlian photography (Kp), gas discharge visualization (GDV), and polychromatic interference photography (PIP). This paper explores such claims and argues that the images produced can be explained by employing concepts drawn from the physical sciences. It is suggested that techniques such as KP, GDV, or PIP currently offer inadequate reliable research evidence concerning their application as diagnostic or imaging alternatives. Consequently, their clinical use is subject to dispute. Kirlian photography and its derivatives may, however, be useful as a research tool by providing visual records of complex bodily responses to experimental situations (Duerden 2004).

In 1939, Semyon Kirlian was invited to fix an electrotherapy instrument in an academic laboratory. While engaged in fixing, he found out that when a patient underwent treatment with the instrument, very small light sparkles were produced between the electrodes. He tried to take photos of the light but understood that recording the event is possible even without a camera. He discovered that if he holds a film between his hand and the high-frequency sparkles, a shining image of his fingers is developed. Other living materials also made images, which were granulated with spots and stains, while lifeless materials could not make any image. Kirlian made a machine to produce a high-frequency electrical field that between its two electrodes two hundred thousand sparkles were produced in each second. He also designed a light window to make direct observation of the process possible (Leonidov 1962).

According to Kirlian, the signals of inner status of the living organism are reflected in brightness, darkness, and color of flames. The activities of inner life of human are written in this light hieroglyph. Until now, we have made an instrument to record this hieroglyph, but further research is needed to decode it (Ostrander & Schroeder 1984).

Kirlian and his wife worked on their instrument and completed it with the aid of specialists of different disciplines until 1964 in which a new horizon was opened up to this field of research. The results of their studies demonstrated that all living organisms have a frame of energy which is similar to body in shape, but it is rather independent from the body. By using their camera, they took a photo of a leaf. Then they cut one third of the leaf and took another photo. A short while after cutting a part of the leaf, the image of that separated part remained as a phantom and the whole image of the leaf was retained. This finding can explain the phantom phenomena or imaginary limb in patients, who had a limb amputation but report some sensations from that limb.

A group of biophysicists and biochemists are studying the energetic limbs by electron microscopy in Kirov State University in Almaty. They have stated that these limbs are "made of a sort of primitive plasma, which is made from ionized particles. This feature is not discrete and irregular and has a unified mechanism" and can be called "biological plasma body." (ibid)

Gas discharge visualization (GDV) was proposed by Konstantin Korotkov in the 1990s. Another GDV subtype is the monopulse plasmagraph (MP) developed by Vadim Bondarev. Both approaches lend themselves to research evaluation. However, concerns about validity and reliability of such devices remain (Bell et al. 2003).

Certain proponents of the GDV and MP systems have developed computer-based analysis that claim to provide detailed whole-body diagnostic information from variations in fingertip discharge patterns.

Whilst an interesting concept, it is difficult to understand how clinically meaningful information can reliably be generated using this technique (Duerden 2004).

PIP was developed by Harry Oldfield. This technique administers a computer-processed video image that claims to highlight the body's energy field, the acupuncture energy lines (meridians), and midline energy centers (chakras). The colors and patterns produced are then analyzed according to their location over or around the body. These are then correlated to the aura, chakras, and meridians, thus informing diagnosis and treatment. The colors are chosen by the software designer and so are arbitrary. Zones of contrast are observable in clothing and shadows as much as the subject's body. It is therefore questionable whether validity and reliability can be given to any diagnosis based on such images.

An interesting finding about plasma is the fact that the only thing that can effectively sustain plasma is a magnetic field. With regard to the electromagnetic field of the body, it is possible to assess and measure the field precisely and quantitatively with the aforementioned instrument. Consequence of these findings culminated in the achievement of some certain precise diagnostic methods to evaluate body energetic fields which, along with other diagnostic systems, can provide accurate evaluation of diseases (see Ostrander & Schroeder 1984).

Employing these diagnostic techniques that are widely used in many clinics of complementary medicine and energy therapy (except for the SQUID that few centers hold it because of its expensiveness) enables us to have objective evaluations of interventions or bioenergy, energetic disorders, and also the energetic changes following the intervention. It is noteworthy. It is worth mentioning that semiology of these changes is under development, and these signs have not been decoded completely, and in many cases, they are at the experimental stage.

Subjective Diagnostic Techniques

Compared with the objective methods, in subjective methods instead of using instruments, measurement depends on cognitive, sensory, and extrasensory abilities of the users and natural and real atmosphere, and paying attention to context of the environment is preferred to the laboratory environment. However, these methods are not as reliable, valid, and precise as the quantitative methods. In general, these methods are more flexible and try to give interpretational explanation of the events, although, as regards the context and holistic view of these methods, they are more compatible with the theoretical and philosophical basis of energetic approaches. These two objective and subjective methods can be considered in a single continuum, and it is better to use them in a joint manner.

Many energy therapists claim that they are able to scan the energetic fields of people by hand and diagnose the disorders, and, of course, they suggest some methods to learn these skills (Luebeck 1991; Watson 1999). Some studies have verified the information obtained in this way (Oschman 2000a).

In some of the bioenergy-based therapies such as therapeutic touch and healing touch, hands-off scanning of the biofield and diagnosis of depletion (bioenergy deficit), congestion (bioenergy accumulation) and distortion (bioenergy maldistribution), and the location of these disturbances has an important role in the healing process (Hurwitz 2001; Levin & Mead 2008). These practitioners endeavor to invigorate their electromagnetic sensibility and bioenergy-pattern recognition. Both practitioner and client pay attention to the scanning experience in the moment, and healee's feedbacks can be another information resource. But, generally, bioenergy healing is a non-diagnostic management and does not look for pathology. Wholeness, holistic approach, and whole-person equilibrium are the fundamental concepts of it.

According to Mollon (1991), there are delicate energetic systems in our body that can be designated "human aura" or "energy fields." This system is in fact the unconscious source of memories and emotions. Countertransference in psychotherapy can be explained with this theory. In other words, the intuitional views rendered accessible by the therapists' delicate biofield, and some information is constantly, repeatedly transferred between the therapist and the client unconsciously and nonverbally.

Many studies have been carried out on the clinical value of the subjective and intuitive diagnostic method (Tornatore & Tornatore 1977; West 1997). It usually seems uncommon for a specialized physician to understand the individual's health information by analyzing human biofield, as a physician on the ground of his knowledge knows that these signals are beyond the frequency of the five senses.

It is possible that there are other senses that medical textbooks have neglected.

All of us are sensitive to some physical forces around us, and there are apparently some ways to fortify the sensitivity. One of these fortifying methods, which have been used for more than five thousand years, is "radiesthesia."

In this method, the radiesthesists discover the presence of water, metal, etc., under the ground by using a bifurcated or two L-shaped metallic stick. He uses the stick and comprehends their tiny vibrations that are not comprehensible normally in an unconsciousness state. The mechanism of radiesthesia resembles the traditional and subjective diagnosis methods of energy therapists in many respects. Many experiments have been conducted on the reliability and validity of this method in academic centers, and all have testified to its possibility.

Tromp (1968), the Dutch geologist, has demonstrated that radiesthesists are usually sensitive to the earth's magnetic field and react to that much of the field changes that can be measured by magnetometer. The radiesthesists, which were tested for the first time in Physics Laboratory of Paris, could easily detect the electrical current being connected or disconnected by moving behind a coil and holding the radiesthesia stick (Watson 1999). It was demonstrated in Hall University experiments that the blood pressure and pulse rate of radiesthesists increase in some fields (Ostrander & Schroeder 1984). Watson believed that expert radiesthesists are able to work without any instruments.

It is apparent that there are senses other than the commonly known five senses (Oschman 2000a). Murchie (1979) named thirty-two other senses or sensory windows. He maintained that many people are able to hear the radar waves, which are electromagnetic signals. Furthermore, the ability to trace cosmos waves has been proved (Guy et al. 1975).

Although these findings bear witness to the existence of such abilities, they raise the question whether they are unique and individual dependent.

The mechanism of energy and information transfer in the body is the same as hitting a billiard ball directly. Signal molecules are scattered by the hit and shake until short-range electrostatic forces (two to three times as large as the molecule size) absorb them and just the same as the time a key in a lock finds the chance to reach the receptor site. In energetic models, biological regulations provide the link between signal and receptor molecules that are not in contact with each other. The term *molecular signals* has an electromagnetic meaning (Benveniste; Smith 1987; Smith & Best 1989). In living organisms, long-range electromagnetic fields send the message to far molecules up to as far as the expanse of their spectrum allows. This finding can to some extent justify the sensitivity and capability of individuals in energetic diagnosis. Smith (1987; Smith & Best 1989) and Benveniste (1998) believe that energetic sensitivity and abilities are not limited to specific individuals, as electromagnetic signaling plays a prominent role in all living organisms.

It seems that the claims of energy therapists, regarding intuitional diagnosis, are defendable from practical as well as theoretical point of view. Subjective diagnostic methods are not as reliable as qualitative methods because of their dependence on proficiency of the therapist in diagnosis and the extent of therapist's sensitivity to electromagnetic fields as well as familiarity with basic sciences of medicine and psychology. However, if the proficiency of the therapist in diagnosis and developing a deep relation between the therapist and the client is confirmed, it can play an important role in treatment. Using these subjective methods in an integrative health system features as a clue for further objective evaluations (Goli 2008).

Salutogenesis versus Pathogenesis

Medicine encountered a drastic turn in the nineteenth century by growth of anatomy and pathology. The reductionistic experiments of Bichat spatialized and localized diseases and developed a methodology to evaluate the static bodies and a large amount of dissective-descriptive information of embodied the diseases (see Foucault 1994). The attitude of biomedicine made diseases and death the foundation of medical and pathological comprehension and anatomical-therapeutic instructions extricated human from his natural life context. Consequently, the organic relationship of human and natural life became more disturbed, incompatible, and quantitative (Goli 2003a and 2003b).

We cope with two principles in pathology of energetic approaches:

First, the principle of normality and abnormality, the biomedicine view tries to discriminate these two entities by presenting various viewpoints such as pathological, statistical, cultural, idealistic views (Dadsetan 1997). Biopsychosocial medicine, by surpassing the boundaries of mind-body dualism conflict, has given a goal to medicine that is the definition of normality and abnormality in spectrum or continuum of health (Goli 2004).

The orthodox view (of biomedicine) simply identifies only two states of normality (health) and abnormality (disease) and treats an individual only as healthy or ill. In this view, the concept of health is static and, of course, ideal.

However, new viewpoints consider abnormality (illness) and normality (health) to have some degrees in health continuum that ranges from death to the complete physical, psychological, spiritual, and social well-being. Each person is at a specific point of the continuum and a biological change (physiological aspect), a wrong belief, thought, behavior (cognitive-behavioral aspect), or even energy disturbance (energetic aspect) may alter the individual's position in the continuum. So an individual is at a specific point in the health continuum whether medicine considers him healthy or ill, and the only systematic and effective action is to move toward the clearest point of the continuum or "higher health" (Goli 2008).

Regarding this, pathology and treatment finds another meaning in health continuum. From a systemic but conservative viewpoint, the task of pathology, in this new model, is to seek indications of homodynamic disturbances in all the levels of biopsychosocial organization; furthermore, it is solelywithin such a network that chemical and physical treatments can effect a sustainable health promotion.

According to a holistic and health-oriented approach, healing is not pathological-based, but is organized around the concept of salutogenesis.

To some trends of healing such as therapeutic touch or Reiki, healing is an "intervention" done by healers—a therapeutic modality imparted by a practitioner to a client. To others, healing is an outcome, such as recovery from illness or curing of a disease. As a result of treatment, whether conventional or alternative, we hope to experience a healing. To some others, in a keen contrast, healing is a "process"—for example, Antonovsky's concept of "salutogenesis manifestly instances the issue." When the pathogenic process is halted, we then, ideally, may begin healing—moving from a state of disease to a state of renewed health (Levin, adapted from Levin & Mead 2008).

The most fundamental rethinking of the pathogenic orientation of Western medical practice and biomedical science is found in Antonovsky's concept of salutogenesis. This concept, he explained, is not just the flipside of pathogenesis—not just oriented to affecting "backward" movement through the natural history of disease, if that were even possible—rather, it is something radically different. Salutogenesis means the creation of health, or the fostering of healing, much as pathogenesis refers to breeding or development of disease. Through the concept of salutogenesis and his subsequent research and writing on the topic, Antonovsky purported to convey a fundamental point: Those factors that initiate and facilitate healing are not necessarily the reverse or negation of those factors that cause disease. For example, tobacco smoking may be a significant risk factor for lung cancer, and obesity may be etiologic for coronary artery disease, but once advanced cases of these diseases have taken hold, we would not expect smoking cessation or weight loss by themselves to cause a malignant tumor to disappear or occluded arteries to unclog, respectively. Healing, in this context, clearly requires something more (Levin & Mead 2008).

This model of the natural history of health provides a salutogenic lens to conceptualize the healing process. It identifies the pathways and constitutes biobehavioral and psychosocial touchstones, along which a diseased person or morbid population must ideally travel in pursuit of health and restoration of wholeness. This model is presumably universal. That is, it operates irrespective of classes of therapeutic interventions or putative physiological mediators. Whether induced and explained by respective methods and mechanisms found in biomedicine, psychosocial therapies, bioenergy-based practices, nonlocal healing (such as purported by paranormal healers), and even the supernatural interventions believed in by the religiously devout, healing comes about through an observable sequence of events that are grounded in the capability of human beings to comprehend, manage, and successfully cope with challenges and threats, thus marshaling the body's innate resources for restoring equilibrium and strengthening resistance (Levin 2003).

Holistic approaches place the individual in a context of dynamic relationship between various aspects of life and environment (Astin 1998), while Western biomedicine tends to focus on a part of the person and elicit a set of signs and symptoms from a unique biopsychosocial matrix. This difference, the philosophical and cultural difference, is the concept of health in the East and the West (Nield-Anderson & Ameling 2000).

By the health continuum and salutogenesis, as basic concepts of healing and also the personal and qualitative concept of illness in pathology of bioenergetic approaches, it can be concluded that:

a) The concept of "disease," as it is considered in the biomedicine viewpoint, does not exist in holistic medicine. Alternatively, the concept of "illness" or the individual's feeling and perception (individual's mental experience) and his cultural and social context are considered in the holistic approach.
b) The "treatment" concept, as it is used in medicine, does not exist in holistic approaches. Because these approaches are person-oriented rather than being disease-oriented and to modify the individual's lifestyle and evolve the person's totality (healing).
c) Healing is based on salutogenesis; a systemic, consciousness-based response of whole person to illness condition.

This is the reason why Reiki teachers consider the healing to be "wisdom" not "treatment," and, accordingly, healing is not a paradigmatic term, but a life-oriented concept.

As it was mentioned before, etiology and pathology of bioenergetic approaches are based on the obstruction of various pathways of bioenergy and incoordination in activities of energy centers, and most of bioenergy-based therapies are non-diagnostic and non-pathologic, but in some of the therapies, the healer has to recognize the pattern and location of bioenergy disturbances.

Certain challenges present in the energy field are commonly encountered by energy practitioners. These include energy depletion, distortion, and congestion. A *depletion* in the energy field adverts to a deficiency of energy in a particular region of the field, which may manifest itself on multiple layers. A *distortion* of the energy field is characterized by an area in which energy is present but not evenly distributed, as it otherwise would be in a balanced energy field. It has a quality of nonregularity. *Congestion* in the energy field refers to an obvious excess of energy, or blockage in the flow of energy, located in a particular region of the field, which again can evince itself on multiple layers. This understanding of bioenergetic pathophysiology is strongly informed by perspectives on nosology and pathology. But this taxonomy also recapitulates concepts pervasive throughout systems and schools of esoteric healing, in general, which consistently implicate congestion and imbalance (akin o this model's distortion) as markers or indicators of disease (Levin 2008).

In explaining the etiology and diseases from bioenergy systems point of view, McKenzie (1998) believes that meridians contain pathways of (bioenergy) current that can be discovered. These pathways are extended throughout the connective tissues (living matrix) (Hover-Kramer 1996). Chakras, which are the focal points in energetic body, are in a higher vibration level than the physical body. Therefore, they can function as the pacemakers of physical events. Regarding this, impairment of the function of these points will cause chemical and physical disorders in the body.

D'Aprile (2002) believes that imbalance in energy current can result in disorder. According to Kim (1995), disturbances in biofield are a pattern of disharmony in which the "Ki" became imbalanced, obstructed, or vitiated. Exhaustion is a sign of in level of "Ki" and, furthermore, complete absence of Ki culminates in death.

As it was mentioned before, in psychoanalysis, energy is more often used to define the etiology of psychological disorders and impaired psychodynamics. Nevertheless, various clinical and laboratory findings have demonstrated that etiology of energetic approaches, which is based on the obstruction of meridians or imbalance of energy foci, is tenable to a great extent (see Oschman 2000a). Various cases or records of biofield disturbances before any clinical and laboratory manifestation on the one hand, and reappearance of signs and symptoms after a dormancy phase on the other hand, are consistent with emphasis of these approaches on the crucial role of bioenergetic balance in physical health (Duerden 2004).

Healing Versus Treatment

In general, therapeutic energetic interventions can amend the imbalance of energy current, improve symmetry, and reestablish free energy current. These interventions are based on the following presumptions:

1) Energy flows inside and around human body.
2) Each person is encircled with a bioenergy field.
3) The bioefield is dynamic. It moves and flows.
4) The biofield can be received. The ability to receive bioenergy is an acquirable skill.
5) Many anecdotal records confirm a cumulative effect of biofield experience, and most of the healees indicate that the bioenergy sensations are more intense during the second healing session (Mansour, Beuche, Laing, Leis & Nurse 1999).
6) Disturbance or imbalance of the human biofield of a person links with his/her illness.
7) Regular reconstruction of biofield restores the individual's balance and develops an environment in which the healing process takes place.
8) Individual biofield is incorporated in a universal field.
9) The patient and the therapist are not separated from each other. Moreover, they are linked and attuned with the universal energy field.

In the chapter entitled "mechanisms," objective and scientific evidence to assess and confirm the above-mentioned hypotheses were provided. Here, we only review these hypotheses. A short look at these concepts reveals that this view is not only a systematic and holistic view to health, but is also more coordinated and compatible with the lifeworld. Moreover, people are more emotionally attuned with this view over health than the method which considers the person as mechanical body with organic injuries. Moreover, considering a more active role for patients in treatment is another reason for acceptance of these therapeutic methods. In addition to these emotional attunements, different clinical studies have substantiated the effectiveness of these energetic approaches to health.

As it was mentioned above, except the trigger-point methods such as acupuncture which have a topological template based on acupoints and meridians, in bioenergy healing, the anatomical pathology is not the basis of diagnosis and treatment. On the other hand, human biofield as a holographic image of whole person is considered, and the goal of treatment is stimulation of salutogenesis and intra/inter/transpersonal biofield coordination rather than removing the pathogenesis. It is clear that this non-diagnostic and communicative management is a person-oriented rather than a disease-oriented approach. Therefore, token (disease)-token (treatment) indication is not sensible and bioenergy conduction to disturbed energy foci is administered by servomechanisms. These interventions usually do not interfere with human organism self-organization and only facilitate the actualization process.

My clinical experiences, in agreement with experiments of many other mind-body practitioners (e.g., Benson 1976; 1997), demonstrate that the efficacy of these methods are more related to personal characteristics and communication of healer/healee (intra/inter/transpersonal factor) rather than the type or severity of the disease. However, the aforementioned findings demonstrate that psychophysical bioenergy healing methods can treat the diseases via the following general effects:

1. Psychoneuroimmunological modulation: Modifying wound healing, autoimmunity, and metaplasia.
2. Stress reduction and catharsis: Improvement in psychological and psychophysical disorders.
3. Coordination with self, other, and universe: Amelioration of spiritual and social welfare.

However, many studies illustrate the correlation of intention with psychophysical variables (Fiol & O'Connor 2004; Nelson 1999; Schlitz 2004). Intentionality gives shape and orientation to these general effects and leads to specific effects. The fundamental principle of healing as intra/inter/transpersonal communicative specificity, the specific effects, is mediated by the specificity of healing intention and healing communication and presence experience rather than the specificity of the treatment method.

Moreover, as it was mentioned in chapter 3, direct and indirect suggestions that are usually induced in treatment process can lead to specific effects. Examples of clinical applications of bioenergy-based therapies noted in chapter 1 were given as clinical guideline for usage of complementary alternative approaches, especially in chronic disorders rather than absolute indications.

Bioenergy Economy

Economy, etymologically, means house management and, generally, means the efficient use of resources. Its basic concepts are production, distribution, consumption, balance, and temperance. Jacobson (1978) defined two fundamentals law of energy economy in the sensory-motor level:

1. The minimum of tensions in the muscles, which is indispensable for an act.
2. Relaxation of other muscles.

Freud described libidinal economy, as that which indicates adaptive control of libido as a psychosomatic energy and consideration of various patterns of dynamism. Reich, by advancing the concepts of the organic energy and sexual economy, and following him, Lowen, by expanding their scope, extended these concepts to the body psychotherapy and bioenergetics framework as a psychosomatic approach to health (Reich 1974; Staunton 2002).

Based on this historical background of application of the concept economy in psychosomatic approach, I have coined the term "bioenergy economy." Economy in this term not only designates the relationship between mind and body, but also cogently affirms the linkage between diagnosis and treatment and medicine and life. In this definition, the bioenergy economy can be considered as a meta-cognitive pattern that reigns over matter, consciousness, and information conversion and transformation in human conditions.

In other words, by being cognizant of the pure bioenergy consumption pattern for subjective and objective tasks and minimizing the false and ineffective investments as well as developing the awareness of subjective and objective resources of bioenergy, we can promote physical, mental, social, and spiritual actualization of ourselves.

As such, bioenergy economy can provide all-encompassing and unique pattern for incorporation and employment of various forms of energy-based therapies. Moreover, it is considered as a common theoretical and clinical foundation for holistic medicine.

Bioenergy economy does not work on the ground of diagnostic classifications as it is not disease-oriented. It is a synthetic and person-oriented method that deals with the openness of energy pathways and biopsychosocial balance.

Regarding this, interventions of this approach are also considered conscious and perspicacious conducting of material-energy-information-knowledge flow in intra/inter/transpersonal spaces and not "treatment." It will be elucidated how these economic strategies can be applied to self and others via environmental, personal, cognitive, behavioral, and bioenergetic interventions. Bioenergy economy is the feminine aspect of health services, which, to a great extent, obviates the need for analytical, more expensive and more invasive interventions. As the definition of bioenergy economy implies, this approach is commonly implicated in the field of "care." In this point of view, care is not used in its masculine biomedicine system definition, but it is the treatment of the dynamism of the disease (not the symptoms) that can cure the psychological and physical disorders solely or in conjuction with analytical treatments. However, its main goal is self-actualization and consciousness evolution.

In the following part, five levels of bioenergy economy constitutes a model to introduce an integrating bioenergetic approaches into health system and determining the distinct levels of objectives and services and founding a consistent and consolidated system.

The Levels of Bioenergy Economy

Most of the studies in energy medicine focus on hands-on/off and also distant interventions of bioenergy-based healing systems. However, as it was mentioned before, bioenergy healing response is not only a result of local bioenergy emissions, but also it can be motivated and/or fascinated via biorhythms modification, cognitive-behavioral interventions, environmental modulation, and nonlocal interventions. There is no single "life force" or "healing energy." Instead, there are numerous energetic systems in the living body and multitude ways of influencing them. The "living state" and "health" result from the totality of these systems, functioning collectively and cooperatively. As such, diseases and disorders disturb bioenergy flows. When integrated with the discoveries of bodywork, bioenergy, and movement therapists, these concepts can enable energetics to take its proper place in the medicine of the future (Oschman 1998).

These five fields of interventions (figure 5.4) can be employed in an integrative bioenergy-based approach. Each of the bioenergy-based therapies concentrates on some fields, and the others are ignored. In order to establish a bioenergy economy model, we require a multidimensional care and cure program that involves all of these interventional fields in an integrative health system. In the ensuring section, we will expand on the five fields of intervention in bioenergy-based healing response.

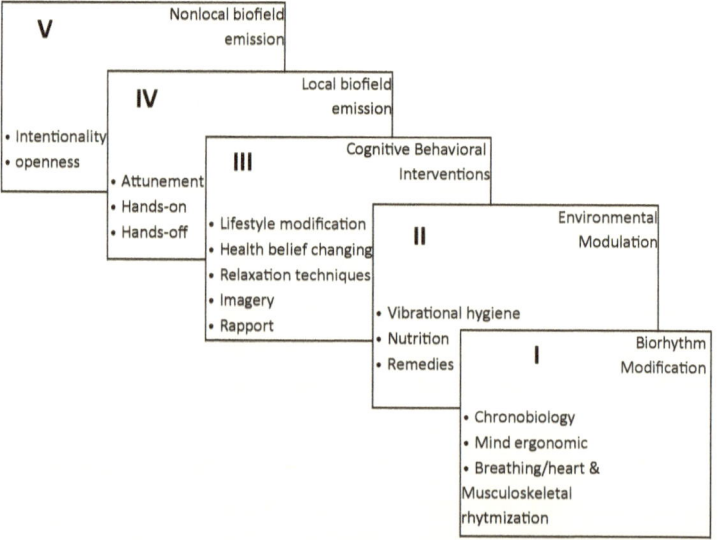

Figure 5.4. Five levels of bioenergy economy for biofield reorganizing and health promotion. This diagram shows all of the conservative interventions that can be employed in an integrative bioenergetic approach to health.

1. Biorhythm Modification

From a vibrational viewpoint, nature is nothing but rhythmical vibrations, and life in this vibrational context has its special rhythms, which are named biorhythms. Chronobiology and mind ergonomy are two related domains of modern knowledge that scrutinize chronological pattern of mind-body activities and suggest appropriate time for each type of performance (Dunlap, Loros & Decoursey 2003; Weeks 2001).

Some of the biorhythm modifications can be classified under the cognitive-behavioral interventions such as breath trainings that change the respiration rhythms and modify the ANS and blood pH and so enhance potential stream and rhythmic musculoskeletal movements (as yogasana, tai chi) via piezoelectric effects provoke and amplify the human biofield.

The electromagnetic rhythms of heart also can be modified intentionally. Various practices that intentionally focus one's attention on the area of the heart, while evoking sincere feelings of love and appreciation, lead to a more regular variation in heart rate, a condition the authors refer to as coherence. This regular variation reflects a balance and coherence between the heart rate and the rhythms of the two branches of the autonomic nervous system, the sympathetic and parasympathetic that regulate heart rate (Oschman 1998).

The heart harmonies not only can change ANS balance, but also can change DNA and genetic activities. A relationship between DNA and heart coherence has been hinted at by work of Rein and McCraty (1993). Their model involves the well-documented ability of DNA to act as a resonant antenna. The authors suggest that the DNA, throughout the body, both receives and transmits information encoded in the heart's electrical rhythms and in the oscillations of the DNA molecule itself.

What has been obscure about the model of Rein, McCraty, and others is the precise mechanism by which the heart rhythms interact with DNA. The resonant properties of DNA molecules, such as the response of DNA to pulsing magnetic fields, have been well documented (e.g., Pienta & Coffey 1991; Liboff et al. 1984; Takahashi et al. 1986). Moreover, it has recently been discovered that DNA molecules have a tendency to pack together in a crystalline array (Peterson 1997), which affects their resonance.

Modification, in aforementioned biorhythms, is an effective way to promote bioenergy economy and health.

2. Environmental Modulation

In addition to internal biorhythms, there are several external rhythms that can affect human organisms. Some studies indicate significant coherence between solar (Gifford 2007; Groome 2001; Pengelley & Asmundsen 1971; Randler 2009), lunar (Discepolo 2009), and Schumann resonances (Sentman 1995), rhythmic alternations, and mind-body modalities. Organizing the life schedule in accordance with these external rhythms may be a useful measure in the bioenergy economy direction. Geomagnetic micropulsations and geopathic stress, as terrestrial variations, can alter physical and mental parameters. Alterations or permutations in the worksite and bedplace, in addition to other architectural and geographical considerations, can be useful for primary and secondary prevention of health-related problems (e.g., Bell et al. 1996; Gifford 2007; Jacobs 1987; Jacobson 1978; Miller 1998; Randler 2009).

Purification, modification, and improvement of artificial fields, especially fifty to sixty cycle-power signals, as well as microwaves and other radio frequencies are other measures to optimize biofield and effect a healthy state (Becker 1990; Oschman 2000a).

Vibrational medicines, like homeopathic remedies, should be classified as environmental modulation because these remedies are adopted and potenized natural substances that prescribed for special health states. In fact, homeopathic remedies are energy-information formulas with their special vibrational signatures. Therefore, it can be considered as selective environmental vibrations (Carlston 2006).

In traditional medicine, especially Hippocratic medicine and ayurveda, foods are not only metabolisms' raw material, but can also modify the humors and bioenergy because of their special nature. They believe that components, composition, and the manner of preparation of food determine its qualitative and energetic effect (Frawley 1997).

In Taittiriya Upanishad, the energetic and ontic relationships between human and food is considered thus:

I am food, I am the eater of food, I eat the eater of food, I consume the entire universe. My light is like the sun (ibid).

Many of the healing traditions underscore the importance of moral, spiritual, and natural aspects of nutrition, since they believe that food is the capacitor of its vital force and so is the initial biofield of both provider and user.

There is no sufficient evidence for these hypotheses, but it seems that these considerations can be useful for mental and spiritual fitness of both healer and healee.

3. Cognitive-Behavioral Interventions

As mentioned before, all of the bioenergy-based therapies contain cognitive-behavioral elements, some of which are necessary to facilitate bioenergy motivation and transference. These cognitive-behavioral motifs are: Passive concentration and guided imagery.

Passive concentration is the preliminary attitude of each relaxation technique, and relaxation response is usually provoked in bioenergy healing process. "Be open to" and "let it be done" are the common attitudes of healers and healees and the crux of bioenergy healing.

Passive concentration paves the way for healing imagery, which is guided directly and/or indirectly and finally changes the psychoneuroimmunological programming.

Concentrating passively on bioenergy exchanges and imagining the bioenergy flow and healing process are two mental activities, which are employed in bioenergy-based techniques by both healer and healee, either consciously or unconsciously.

In transpersonal psychology, different symbols and shapes are used for imagining, ranging from the intrapersonal to the transpersonal, which are all applied to bring about changes in the dynamics of psyche and body. Based on the studies by Gerard and Watkins, Rowan categorized the symbols that are used for therapeutic purposes into the three groups—controlled symbolic visualization, spontaneous symbolic visualization, and symbolic visualization for psychospiritual development (Ferrucci 1983; Rowan 2005).

In controlled symbolic visualization, specific symbols such as mandalas and yantras, sun, or crystals are used to guide attention and induce related changes.

In spontaneous symbolic visualization, mind is allowed to give an imaginary and symbolic shape to an internal perception of an emotion like anger or a symptom like pain. Hence, in a self-motivated manner, mind would be activated and by symbolization of that experiment will get familiar with its unknown aspects and the ability to exert control over the experiment is increased.

In symbolic visualization for psychospiritual development, mind is oriented toward the internal wisdom and inspiration, moral concepts, and spiritual values. Its aim is to actualize these issues and spiritual values and consequently occasion personality evolution (Rowan 2005).

Furthermore, these motifs in some of the techniques, such as prayer or Reiki II, III, can be employed only by healer, and several studies on nonlocal healing corroborate this fact (see, e.g., Schlitz 2004; Schlitz & Braud 1997).

Other cognitive-behavioral interventions—such as brief cognitive-behavioral therapy (CBT), physical trainings, and also lifestyle modifications—are recommended in some of the bioenergy healing systems.

An appropriate planning for integrating bioenergy-based therapies comprises two dimensions. The first one is considering all physical, mental, energetic, and spiritual parameters; and the second one is simplifying the health promotion packages in order to increase the acceptance chance and decrease failures and time/money expenditure.

Reframing, refocusing, and remodeling of lifestyle and so contributing some certain new elements, such as meditation, can be cost-effective and applicable to health behavior change and psychoneuroimmunologic modulation.

4. Local Emissions

Some of the bioenergy-based techniques, like the therapeutic touch, are based on bioenergy awareness and training, but others like Reiki are based on attunement for initiation and harmonizing the healee's biofield. Attunement is a sort of healing presence in which a biofield pattern—as a resonant, healthy blueprint—is transferred to another person and entrains his/her biofield.

In hands-on techniques, hands are in contact with skin and establish an intimate healer—healee communication, but in some it may include resistance in the client. Anyhow, because of moral considerations, clinical limitations, and psychological variations, we may prefer to employ hands-off techniques.

In addition to the aforementioned indications, some of the healers and schools of healing underline the advantages of hands-off techniques, including more powerful perception of bioenergy flow and psychological (Qikinetic effects) and physical (Qidynamic effects) inductions.

In some bioenergy healing systems, such as Reiki, healing, or self-healing, training starts with hands-on method, then proceeds with hands-off method, and finally results in nonlocal healing (Stein 2000).

Geggus (2004) introduced four kinds of touches, which are employed in bioenergy healing systems. These are blending, streaming, meridianing, and interface (figure 5.5). This classification can be wielded in an integral bioenergy healing approach.

Blending occurs where both people merge at the point of contact so that a part of them becomes a whole which belongs neither to the one or the other, but a mélange one nor the other but both. This naturally tends to happen if contact is prolonged. In streaming, the energy of one person flows into the other. In meridianing, a person acts as a conduit for ushering an energy that emanates from outside. Interface touch is a contact that consciously maintains the boundaries between the two people are aware. Thus, they remain very sensitively "in touch" and yet distinctly separate.

Many skilled therapists are not conscious of whether they are blending, streaming, meridianing, or at interface. This can make it hard for them to be clear, consistent, and energetically accurate as to the kind of connection they make with their clients (2004).

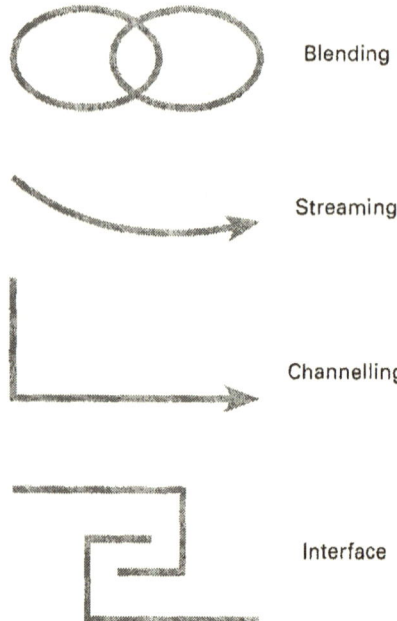

Figure 5.5. The four kinds of touch that may be used to work with energy (quoted from Geggus 2004, With permission from Elsevire)

According to a traditional view, these energetic interventions can be performed with any of the following bodies with defined limits (Baginski, Sharamon, Hanslian, Baker & Harrison 1997).

a) Elemental body
b) Energetic and etheric body (about twenty centimeters of the skin surface)
c) Mental body (up to two and a half meters of the skin)
d) Wisdom body (up to six meters of the skin)

5. Nonlocal Emissions

We discussed about evidences and probable mechanisms of distance healing before. These studies display the effects of the specific intentions by one person and the concurrent measurement of physiological parameters in another person without any sensorimotor and local communication (see ch. IV).

Several kinds of nonlocal communication are in bioenergy-based therapies. These healing relations can be mediated by verbal (prayer), contemplative (healing meditation), imagery, symbolic (Reiki III) and/ or iconic tools. These nonlocal media can harmonize, synchronize, and direct intentions and biofield toward the absent target. In prayer, for instance, a religious phrase or any sort of self-talk is repeated, while the individual believes in an omnipresent and omniscient responsive network or existence.

Healing meditation, as a contemplative healing technique, is different from relaxation and imagination. Healing meditation is initiated by contemplating on a specific intention but continued in a no-mind state and pure witnessing. The presence experience extends initial intention through and beyond the time and space.

Some of the experienced healers prefer to imagine the healing process and healed person, and some others employ mystical symbols in order to facilitate the biofield nonlocal transference. Hon-sha-ze-nen symbol in Reiki is a case in point (see appendix A).

Administration of the healee's image or other related icons works with the same mechanism of voodoo but in the opposite direction. Voodoo can be defined as nonlocal nocebo (Baginski, et al. 1997; Roberts & Groome 2001), and by changing the content to healthy intention it can be a useful technique.

These techniques should be coalesced in a complementary manner in order to produce the best results.

Table 5.6 demonstrates different methods of distant healing. These techniques, which are done via conscious direction of nonlocal emissions, are categorized on the basis of media. Furthermore, the basis (techniques, tools, and presumptions) of these strategies is demonstrated in the table 5.6. Although the classification is rather allegorical and rudimentary, it can be inspiring for both clinical practitioners and researchers.

Nonlocal media	Technique	Tool	Assumption
Verbal	Prayer	Self-talk	Omnipresent intelligent network
Contemplative	Meditation	Initiation	Intention expansion
Imagery	Imagination	Positive images	Imaginal creation
Symbolic	Visualization	Mystic symbols	Mystical relations
Iconic	Focusing	Icons	semiosis

Figure 5.6. Five kinds of nonlocal media and their main techniques, tools, and assumption. This classification emphasizes the characteristic features of each medium, and in fact, there is only a fuzzy distinction between these fields of action.

Aggravation and Recovery of Energetic Disorders

Many therapists as well as the patients or healthy people, who have experienced bioenergy healing, have adverted to experience physical or psychological symptoms transiently following the energetic interventions (Oschman 2000a).

The individuals, who have usually experienced these symptoms, in the course of their lives they reexperience them during the healing process. For instance, if he/she had anxiety or lower back pain a few years ago and now after one or some bioenergy healing sessions, the patient again experiences lower back pain or anxiety even more severe than before. These symptoms, which are called aggravation, are considered as the most important clinical manifestation in all bioenergetic approaches.

In homeopathy, aggravation is regarded as a step in the treatment process rather than a side-effect and is defined as transient worsening or presentation of symptoms. This is interpreted as a good sign and indicates that the vital energy and the healing potential of the patient have responded to the energetic medicine and is in an acceptable level (Riley 2002).

When the vital energy is in a low level, the diseases tend to become hidden or chronic. By upgrading the vital energy, the organism is ready to directly deal with the disorder. So signs and symptoms are presented or worsened at this stage.

A similar phenomenon is manifested in psychotherapy of neurosis. When the individual's ego does not have sufficient energy to confront a tension, via the defense mechanisms it sends it to the unconscious mind. This gradually will turn into anxiety, phobia, depression, psychosomatic, or behavioral disorders (Smith & Broida 2007).

Catharsis and abreaction mechanisms seek to express offences and psychological injuries. This process is usually accompanied by emotional release, transient instability, and impulsive behaviors, and the individual will possibly reexperience that tension severely and transiently. Nevertheless, after this step significant recovery is observed (ibid).

Hence, aggravation can be considered as a deep process of catharsis and abreaction of mind-body and the awakening of body memory because of an energetic stimulus and as a result of improvement in vital energy level.

Four important points should be considered about energy therapists:

First: If the aggravation is ensued by severe physical or psychological symptoms, regarding the possibility of recurrence of the disease especially in elderly or patients with history of debilitating diseases, the patient should be referred to a physician for striking certainty.

Second: During the aggravation, the patient should keep in touch with the therapist or his assistant or at least receive the emotional and physical support from relatives, friends, and/or self-help groups.

Third: If the aggravation lasts more than three to four weeks without relief of the symptoms, medical consultation should be asked.

Fourth: Patients with unstable moods, borderline personality, or with background psychosis will present some symptoms in case of imperative contacts, magical or delusional suggestions, or inappropriate indirect suggestions. These presentations should not be construed as aggravation. They rather arise from inappropriate screening and inappropriate intervention. Moreover, it is evident that it would not result in recovery.

Is Bioenergy Intelligent?

Most trainees and teachers of bioenergy healing systems maintain that the Cosmic Prana and/or bioenergy, which are transferred via the healers, are intelligent currents. Healing this current is usually named after that specific approach. For instance, it is a prevalent idea that "Qi healed him" or "Reiki is the guide." Reiki is in fact the name of the supreme sense that leads the healing stream and life of practitioners.

There are three criticisms to this viewpoint:

First: Considering Reiki or any other method or event as a subject is a kind of animism and enters the delusional suggestions into the individual's life.

Second: If in any bioenergy-based discipline, energetic events are called with a particular jargon and the general effects of energy fields are attributed to its discipline, this may merely result in obfuscation and bewilderment; it will also occasion some social and clinical iatrogenic problems.

Third: Although many physicists believe that the world is made up of consciousness and the consciousness is not in things but it is the things themselves (see Capra 2000), the consciousness that is intended by bioenergy healers and is called Qi, Prana, or Reiki, it in fact refers to and is expressive of the semiconscious sensory-motor as well as psychoneuroimmunolical experiences of the healers and healees (Goli 2008).

In this regard, Oschman (2002), in a conversation with a Reiki master, denotes that from the scientific point of view, the supreme intelligence they talk about is nothing but the inner wisdom and the innate sense that all of us have. When our mental activities reach the relaxation state, we have access to it, and our subconsciousness allows us to organize what has really happened.

He adds that in each second, only a small portion of the eleven-million bits of information, which has reached our brain from senses, are transferred to us via the unconsciousness and are analyzed in the absence of consciousness. Hence, if we trust our assumptions and intuitions, we have trusted the information that is closer to reality than the way we sense reality, because it is based on the information which had more time to be analyzed.

He believes that the injured tissue sends some signals, which induce in the energy system of hands and helps bioenergy practitioners to go to the right place. This theory is worth of testing.

Therefore, this theory, which denotes that the intelligent energy goes where it is needed, is scientifically untenable. Nonetheless, scientific evidence demonstrates that stronger and more harmonic energy fields dominate the weaker and less-harmonic ones according to entrainment phenomenon. Thus, it is evident that bioenergy fields are drawn too assimilated in the positions and fields that are disorganized.

Some trainees and therapists of energy healing have the experience that sometimes without any prior information, during the therapy session, feels that they should transfer more energy to a special position or hands should be stopped on that position in an ideomotor manner and what comes as surprise it was later confirmed that there was a disorder on that special position. In fact, it is the unconscious intelligence of the therapist that via the unconscious sensory-motor feedbacks and on the basis of distinguishing the qualitative field differences of that location, focuses on it. Thus, it is the intelligence of human organism that on the one hand controls the reception, generation, direction, and energy-focus processes (healee's organism) and activates the healing mechanisms and on the other hand diagnoses the energetic disorders (healer's organism) and generates fields proportionate to the need of the organism; occasionally, it even plays all these roles together (Goli 2008).

However, the openness of the individual's bioenergy field to the organized human and cosmos energies as well as the openness of the individual to his unconscious sources are the precondition to the activation of these intelligent processes ancient masters, probably being aware of these mechanisms, employed bioenergy, *Reiki*, *Baraka*, or . . . as metaphors for individual openness. Moreover, there are findings that reveal the specific effects of each of these energetic systems. This, in addition, is indicative of reception and the selective guidance of human organism, and not of the existence of a soul with such characteristics.

So bioenergy intelligence can be considered as the intelligence of healing processes, and this metaphoric description is a way to diminish resistance and disbelief of the individual to these natural and ubiquitous processes in human and the nature.

Ethical Principles

In traditional healing systems, spirituality and ethical fostering are the essential instructions and considerations for the healers to be eligible and competent and even for healees. Opening up to God, universe, and/or the others necessitates ethical principles to establish and maintain definite and distinct boundaries in professional relationships for the protection of client's autonomy and health.

Several associations and institutions of various bioenergy-based disciplines enact their peculiar ethical codes.

These standards, some most prominent and prevalent of which have been enlisted as follows, are common in most ethical rubrics:

Maintaining the professional limits

1- Maintaining the personal boundaries
2- Cost-benefitness of services
3- Emphasis on the active role of clients
4- Scientific and rational illumination of clients
5- Emphasis on the spiritual aspect of life

Biomedical ethics focuses on establishing an appropriate balance between tow philosophical approaches: Paternalism (utilitarianism) and autonomy (existentialism).

Paternalism refers to the established idea of the provider holding special knowledge and skills and using these to help the patient, as a father would care for a child. The principle of benefiting and not harming the patient is the dominant ethical consideration (Brody 1997). This is consistent with the principles of nonmaleficence, beneficence, and a concept of personal virtue. Nonmaleficence is characterized by the following statement: "One ought not to inflict evil or harm" (Beauchamp & Childress 1994).

In contrast, autonomy has been an important approach that underlies decision-making in medical care and has been championed by nursing. Autonomy is the duty to decide responsibly for oneself about one's own interests (Ashley & O'Rourke 1994). Two conditions are essential to this principle—liberty and agency. Liberty refers to independence from controlling influences or constraints, and agency refers to the capacity for intentional action (Wardell & Engebretson 2001).

The focus in health-care delivery is the concern for quality of life in long-term management of chronic illnesses and the importance of lifestyle issues in prevention. This divergence from intensive care management challenges the traditional patient—provider relationship and requires that tilt the locus of responsibility for action toward the patient and out of the exclusive control of the provider (ibid).

This epidemiological shift changes the ethical and finally medical model to a communicative model on the base of lifeworld of clients. Mishler (1981 and 1984) described clinical discourse on the groundwork of the theory of communicative action of Jorgen Habermas (1984). Habermas demonstrates the dialectic of goal-directedness of system rationalization and ethical values of lifeworld rationalization in the medical discourse. This theoretical framework shows technological dominance and blockage and distortion and/or ignorance of ethnicity of lifeworld. More humanistic and effective medical care necessitates a communicative and ethical reform in medical model and establishment of a sustainable equilibrium between paternalism (goal-directed or doing values) and autonomy (being values) in health and healing.

Wardell and Engebretson (2001) present an analytic-qualitative study on ethical codes and standards of three organizations: Healing Touch International (HTI), Reiki Touch Institute of Holistic Health (RT), and American Holistic Nurses Association (AHNA). They characterized several parameters of paternalism and autonomy in the members and ethical codes of these organizations (figure 5.7).

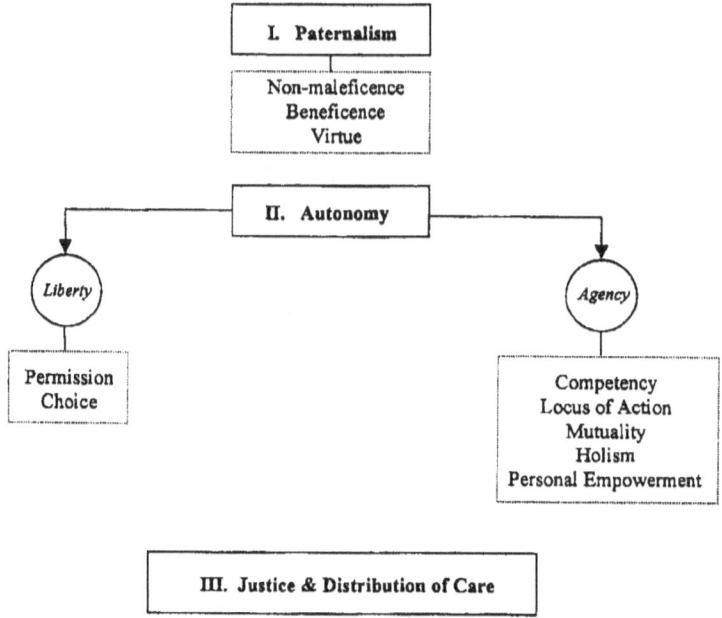

Figure 5.7. Representative ethical approaches and principles in healers

They have worked out several paternalistic parameters and prescriptions from the published codes/standards:

Nonmaleficence: Nonmaleficence—to do no harm—was specifically identified in the HTI and RT documents and implied in the AHNA statements. For example, this statement prohibits the inappropriate use of healing energy: "No energy is given beyond the capacity for the person to receive following the principle: do no harm (HTI)."

Beneficence: Beneficence—to do good—was specifically stated in all three documents and even more frequently implied as the following statements illustrate. "[The] client's plan of holistic nursing care shall be implemented within the context of the system of the individual to progress forward and upward toward a higher potential of functioning (AHNA)." "We agree to touch others . . . with an understanding of the extraordinary power we have in our safe-keeping (RT)."

Virtue: One striking difference between the ethical statements of all three groups and those of traditional biomedical or nursing ethics was the emphasis on the personal virtues of the healer. All addressed the importance of the attitude, intent, and actions of the healer. Statements that reflect this view include the following: "Strive to achieve harmony in your own lives and assist others striving to do the same (AHNA) and our first duty is to heal ourselves: spiritually, mentally, and physically. We realize that we are not only instruments, but also models of healing (RT)." The emphasis on development of the healer is related to the centrality of spirituality in healing.

And so after reviewing and analyzing the codes/standards, several autonomic parameters and prescriptions were derived:

Autonomy, incorporating both concepts of liberty and agency, was well-represented in all three documents. Exemplars will be used to identify how each of these was met.

Two aspects of liberty, client permission and respect for choice, are evident in the following statements: "The individual rights are upheld at all times and the person's coping method is to be respected (HTI) and we will give Reiki when requested—and only when requested (RT)."

Concepts related to agency included client competency, locus of action, mutuality, holism, and personal empowerment. Competency was implied in this statement: "The client is a fully knowledgeable participant in the health/healing process based on his/her ability (HTI)."

Locus of action is related to clients' active participation in healing and is evident in the following statement: "Healing is an individual lived experience. Therefore a healing touch practitioner is a facilitator of the health/healing, not the cause of the changes. Change is within the control of the individual at all times (HTI)."

The relationship between client and provider was described through the concept of mutuality. This statement is expressive of this mutual agreement: "We agree to touch others with . . . an ongoing awareness of their and our spiritual, mental, and physical boundaries (RT)."

The perspective of holism was voiced by the following: "Holistic nurses shall focus care on the whole client . . . not merely the current presenting symptoms or tasks to be accomplished (AHNA)." The inclusion and centrality of the spiritual domain in healing was evident as all documents had several statements honoring the spiritual nature of the client and the healer. Spirituality not only involved the individual client, but also extended beyond the individual to the nature of the work as "holistic nurses shall develop competency in practice to facilitate a sense of sacredness about their work (AHNA)."

Client empowerment was an additional consideration in the ethic of personal agency and was evident in the following statement: "We will encourage them not only to receive the Reiki that is their birthright, but also to claim their personal power to take charge of their own healing (RT)."

At the end of discussion, we introduce "the Canadian Reiki Association Code of Ethics" as a sample of the bioenergy-based healing ethical standard. The eighteenfold ethical principle of CRA is:

1. The health and well-being of the client/student is the prime consideration of the member.
2. The client is entitled to truth, confidentiality, and the respect of their human dignity.
3. The client has the right to accept or refuse any form of treatment.
4. Members shall not refuse a client on the basis of sex, race, religion, sexual orientation, or political belief. However, notwithstanding this clause, members reserve the right to refuse a client for reasons of personal safety and/or other reasons, which do not contravene the aforementioned item.
5. Members should retain accurate and up-to-date records on their dealings with the client. These records should be maintained in a secure location and must be considered confidential. No information contained within the records should be released without the written consent of the client.
6. Members shall dress in a professional manner conducive to the holistic service being provided and be neat and clean in his/her own personal hygiene.
7. Members shall ensure that their professional conduct is beyond reproach. They shall not take physical, sexual, psychological, or

financial advantage of the client. They must not interfere in the clients' personal affairs.

8. Members shall not practice or teach Reiki if they are in any condition, which compromises the quality of their services, such as inebriation, or if their mental faculties are lessened for any reason whatsoever, and they shall never offer liquor to their clients.

9. Members will never ask a client to disrobe and will not allow such action to take place, nor will the member touch the genital area or anal area or the breasts or areola of their client, nor will the client be allowed to touch the practitioner in such a manner.

10. When the client has given permission for "hands-on" therapy, members shall use light hand pressure when placing hands on the client's body. There will never be a need to rub or manipulate any body part. If the client has not given permission for "hands-on" therapy, the member will complete the entire Reiki session with hands above the body at all times.

11. Members shall not refuse or withdraw services without justifiable cause. Such reasons include but are not limited to conflict of interest between the member and the client that jeopardizes the professional relationship or illegal or unjust or fraudulent actions taken or proposed by the client.

12. Members must recognize their limits of competence and must not undertake issues for which they have no training. Members will not claim that Reiki can cure, nor will they diagnose any medical problems or prescribe, nor will they ever advise a client to stop taking medications, unless qualified to do so. When it is in the clients interests, members should refer the client on to another practitioner or organization that has the training appropriate to the client's needs.

13. Members should continually make an effort to improve their knowledge and professional skills. They should also encourage the public to become educated and informed about the practice and teaching of Reiki and about the development of a health-enhancing lifestyle in general.

14. Teaching members should not encourage the practice of Reiki by persons, who are not competent or who have insufficient training

or certification. They should not grant certificates of attendance or competence to anyone whose skills and/or ethical conduct have a valid reason to doubt. Teaching members should report any such cases to the CRA.

15. Members are responsible for reporting any member of the CRA who does not respect this code of ethics. This requirement aims to ensure the protection of the public interest and also to protect the good name and professional reputation of the CRA.

16. Members agree that failure to abide by the terms, conditions, and stipulations of this code of ethics will leave the subject to action, whether legal or other, by the CRA. Action may include but is not limited to: temporary or permanent suspension of membership, public notification of a member's transgression, and/or suspension of membership, legal action. In addition, members understand that breaching any or all of code numbers 7, 8, 9, and 10 will result in immediate termination of their membership.

17. Members acknowledge that a code of ethics cannot cover every case of what is ethical and what is not. Therefore, it is understood that members must behave in accordance with the ethical standards of the province and country in which they reside.

18. It is understood that the CRA is hereby saved harmless from liability of any kind whatsoever for the actions or lack thereof of its registered practitioners and/or registered teachers in fulfillment of their association membership.

The shift in the expression of the principles of beneficence and client agency allowed the healers to employ the therapeutic effects of placebo, suggestion, optimism, hope, and surrender with avoidance of nocebo effects (Wardell & Engebretson 2001).

Chapter VI

Research Methodology of Energetic Approaches

Methodological Principles

In general, two types of energy fields are used in energy medicine:

a) Veritable fields that are precisely measurable.
b) Putative fields that cannot be measured precisely (Berman & Straus 2004).

Bioenergy practitioners normally use putative fields, while veritable fields are used only in treatments that use synthetic sources, which are precise and controllable. Energy fields that are also called "biofields" have a variable and very complex structure. Although the components of these fields are measurable, their complicated interferences and wide-range changes make their accurate measurement, as an interfering therapeutic factor, implausible.

When the body is influenced by a determined, short-frequency synthetic electromagnetic field, we can understand how changes that will happen, for instance in bone marrow regeneration, relate with our independent variable that is the electromagnetic field.

Now, suppose various organs produce electromagnetic fields with different frequencies (fields of different organs such as heart, voluntary muscles, eyes, brain . . .), their frequencies alters in terms of time-place changes as well as emotional, relational, and motional changes. Consequently, the complex interference pattern of these fields, some of which are increasing and some decreasing, will change in accordance with the above-mentioned changes. Now, how can we define the exact effect of this therapeutic intervention on a biological process? Moreover, it should be added to this complex matrix that various organs produce different fields ranging from heat waves and laser waves to plasma mass, which can produce even opposite effects with regard to cognitive, emotional, and behavioral changes of the individual (Goli 2008).

Thus, research in this field has some specific complexities, and many common quantitative methods in biomedicine cannot test and assess the effects of these therapeutic methods.

In many complementary treatments, the complexity of natural treatment factors lead to similar problems. On the other hand, spread and acceptance of complementary and alternative medicine (CAM) in the world especially in Western countries have challenged health researchers. CAM approaches have been expanded in different cultures and possess different diagnostic and therapeutic methods. Therefore, standard and appropriate methods to evaluate all these health and treatment methods have not been developed as yet.

The new challenge of CAM is the way to study and assess hypotheses of these methods. Thus, different organizations and researchers have suggested various research methods with different methodological standards.

Concerning this, World Health Organization (WHO) have strived to develop and promote research methods, and texts of traditional medicine and many researchers have followed this approach until now (WHO 2000).

Generally, traditional, complementary, and alternative medicine (TCAM) have been classified and organized by different authorities with different applications and potentials. According to what was mentioned above, WHO (2000) has classified these approaches in terms of methodological differences. This classification groups these approaches into main categories of procedure-based and remedy-based treatments. Some of the remedy-based treatments are herbal therapy, homeopathy, and ayurveda pharmacology, while yoga, Reiki, and the other bioenergy-based therapies belong to the procedure-based group.

By introducing standard methods of research methodology for remedy-based and procedure-based treatments, WHO has facilitated the opportunity for these treatments to be incorporated in common medical systems. Qualitative studies, which have been carried out extensively in recent years, can appraise many hypotheses of CAM. Development of technologies of the instruments, which measure the biological fields, has contributed to the extension of objective and quantitative studies on bioenergy-based therapies that mainly belong to procedure-based treatments.

Nevertheless, regarding the skill-basedness of these interventions and their dependence on the mind-body state of both of the therapist and clients as well as many complex transpersonal factors, the control of research conditions, repeatability of these studies, and their comparison them with placebo and sham interventions, are rendered hard and even impossible in many cases. Some review studies, which were performed on touch therapy and distance healing in recent years, have indicated their higher validity and reliability, but this is not the case for bioenergy healings that are carried out in the presence of the therapist, and avoiding the bias and controlling the test conditions is difficult (Crawford, Spparber & Janis 2003).

On the other hand, the common theme in integrative medicine (IM) is patient-centered partnering in care between patients and providers. Despite the stated ideal, few studies have scrutinized patients' perspectives on their actual experience in the context of a specific care model (Koithan et al. 2007).

Therefore, the following research methods that are suggested are mainly qualitative methods. However, appropriate fulfillment of these methods has sufficient reliability and validity.

In the ensuing parts, the principles of research methodology of procedure-based bioenergetic therapies will be presented.

General Considerations

To assess the effectiveness of a therapeutic method, one should evaluate and compare it with other treatment methods. WHO (2000) has suggested the following principles for this issue:

- Assessment of the method in terms of its theoretical principles and philosophical framework.
- Assessment of the method in the theoretical framework of biomedicine.

- Comparing the effectiveness of the method with that of other complementary approaches and biomedicine.

Research Literature Review

The primary point for beginning any study is the review and evaluation of previous studies. In cases of lack of written scientific studies, this will be done by studying oral literature and traditional sources. Review of studies enhances the confidence and effectiveness of our current approach and provides evidence for its validity (WHO 2000).

In the two recent decades, systematic experimental studies especially in the frame of PEAR program and nonlocal effects of bioenergy (Jonas & Crawford 2003) as well as *in vitro* studies were carried out (see ch. IV).

A range of so-called target systems has been wielded to study the possible effect of distant intentionality on living systems with a range of possible studies that are nearly as diverse as the processes within an organism that might be influenced. Research participants have included healers, psychics, and unselected laboratory volunteers. The existing literature shows the typical stages of a research paradigm, running the gamut from less to more systematic research over a period of forty years. Despite vast differences in the database of more than 150 studies, the experiments generally fall into two major categories (Shiltz & Braud, 1997).

The first category is a direct analog of actual healing practices. It consists of studies in which a healer seeks to manipulate and mitigate a deleterious process or condition in a target organism. The aim is to improve the organism's vitality or diminish its morbidity. For example, biologist Bernard Grad, a pioneer in this field of study, watered seeds with saline solution that had been treated by a healer and another solution that had not. In a careful, double-blind design, Grad found that the seeds watered with healer-treated saline were more likely to sprout and grow successfully.

Another biologist, Carroll Nash, reported that the growth rate of bacteria could be influenced by conscious intention in controlled, double-blind studies. Likewise, psychological researcher William Braud found a highly significant reduction, attributable to the effect of intention, in hemolysis rates of the participant's own blood cells held in a saline solution in test tubes in a distant room.

Some studies in this category involved an attempt to influence the course of a naturally occurring disease or condition. For example, healers have successfully reduced the growth of cancerous tumors in laboratory animals, which evinced a remarkable reduction in the growth rates in comparison with unhealed control animals. In another example, volunteers successfully minimized complications related to heart disease in hospitalized patients, compared with untreated control patients. It is in this latter case that we find the research that bears the closest resemblance to healing per se (Schlitz & Braud 1997).

A second major category of the impact of distant intentionality on living systems involves the measurement of ongoing normal processes or behaviors in target organisms. The typical experiments are designed to have either neutral or beneficial effects. The research includes effects on long-term factors such as growth of plants or cell cultures and short-term changes in motor behavior or physiological activity. For practical reasons, the study of ongoing normal processes has received the most experimental attention.

In particular, numerous studies have addressed the question of whether physiological measures—specifically autonomic nervous system activity in humans—might be susceptible to distant intentionality. Such measurements as electrodermal activity (EDA) are readily made sensitive indicators and are known to be useful peripheral measures of the activity of the measures that represent a coherent and methodologically consistent subset of overall database studies of the influence of distant intentionality on living systems. What follows is an overview and analysis of this subset of experiments; we have chosen to focus on these experiments because they represent a well controlled and systematic program of study, because there have been heterogeneous replications in numerous laboratories by independent investigators, and because they reside in an area in which the authors have extensive experience (Schlitz & Braud 1997).

In recent years, numerous quasi-experimental (e.g., Denison 2004; Vitale & O'Connor 2006), preexperimental (e.g., Smith & Broida 2007), and also descriptive studies (e.g., Gueldner et al. 2005; Kim 2004; MacNeil 2006) were carried out in the field of bioenergy local effects.

Moreover, there are several systematic studies, meta-analyses, and valuable reports about each bioenergy-based therapies especially Reiki (e.g., Lee, Pittler & Ernst 2008; Tiller 2002), Qigong (e.g., Heron-Marx, Price-Knol, Burden & Hicks 2008; O'Mathuna 2000; Vitale 2007; Winstead-Fry & Kijek 1999), therapeutic touch, (Gallo 2002), energy psychology (e.g., Bell, et al. 2005; Hodge 2007), prayer, and distant healing (e.g., Schlitz 2004).

Crawford and colleagues (2003) believed that this is why research methods are still in their nascent stage, and to achieve this, operational definitions are required. Operational definitions in research clarify the essence of research and increase its reliability and validity. The emphasis on this point is indicative of the importance of being familiar with research methodology for Reiki trainees.

Study Design

Fulfilling a study without having efficient understanding of the pathway and its different steps is not possible. The importance of this issue is the same as the importance of the design for a building, without which a shapeless building will be constructed.

Although the common concepts of clinical research are standard, yet applying them in complementary and energy medicine will lead to new methodological challenges. So WHO (2000) has introduced a range of methods for clinical research in energetic approaches in order to accord more flexibility for this type of research.

a) Single Case Design

This design enjoys many advantages for clinical studies, especially for therapeutic methods and evaluation of illness as it yields a wide range of information. However, such reports are mainly presented by bioenergy practitioners, but they have limitations regarding lack of control of intervening factors and lack of generalization to other circumstances and patients.

Such designs are suitable for development and assessment of clinical fields. For instance, various styles of energetic interventions can be evaluated by this design.

This design does not have control group, but the treatment method can be applied by random.

b) Black Box Design

To research in the field of holistic medicine, black box design can be used. The aim of this design is to separate the therapeutic intervention and its parameters from common clinical situation to avoid it being directed toward a specific treatment package.

Considering this, accurate identification of treatment mechanisms and programs that are not completely controllable and standard is placed in the black box, and the outcome will be studied.

This time-honored method of scientific inquiry is to treat a new phenomenon as a black box whose internal characteristics are unknown but amenable to probe and analysis. One applies some appropriately selected input stimulus (IS) to the box and determines the output response (OR) to the specific stimulus. By varying the IS and correlating the OR with the IS, one deduces information about the most probable behavior of the box for this magnitude of stimulus. One then speculates on models of nature that would first qualitatively and quantitatively reproduce such a spectrum of responses. Then one proceeds to design critical tests for discriminating between the initially acceptable models (Tiller 2002).

Since the true and lawful nature of the box would have a much more complex and rich expression than we could obtain by this limited probing, the exact and complete response function for the box may be characterized by the following general functional form (ibid):

$$\frac{OR}{IS} = f(\varepsilon_1, \varepsilon_2, \varepsilon_3, \ldots, \varepsilon_n; \ x_1, x_2, x_3, \ldots, x_n). \quad (1a)$$

Here, f represents the exact and complete functional relationship between all the possible material parameters, εj, and all the possible experimental variables, Xj, of the system, where unlimited range of magnitude is allowed for these parameters and variables.

Because at any point in time, one has limited cognitive awareness of all these parameters and variables, a limited array of probe stimuli, probe measurement accuracy, financial resources for the probing, and limited patience for endless data gathering, one settles for the following functional expression as the operational response function for the box:

$$\frac{OR}{IS} = f'\left(\varepsilon_1, \ldots, \varepsilon_j; x_1, \ldots, x_j\right) \text{for} \tag{1b}$$
$$\varepsilon_j' < \varepsilon_j < \varepsilon_j''; x_j' < x_j < x_j''.$$

This operational response function, f, involves a limited but sufficient number of parameters and variables with bounded ranges $\left(\varepsilon_j' - \varepsilon_j'' \text{ and } x_j' - x_j''\right)$ for a satisfactory degree of reliability. It is this type of response function that one tries to match with a model so that our successful models simulate idealized nature rather than actual nature.

This is a practical procedure that has been very fruitful for an evolving humanity, and it provides meaningful but relative truth concerning this aspect of nature (Tiller 2002).

This design enables the researcher to assess the effect of holistic treatment methods separated from their own assumptions or biomedicine frameworks.

c) Ethnographic Design

These studies provide documents of the social and cultural texture which bioenergy healing systems have arisen from them and also help us to recognize and interpret the health/illness belifes and behaviors in a specific cultural context. These qualitative methods can maintain primary information from which research hypotheses will be developed or will lead to other studies.

d) Observational Design

Observational studies can maintain many findings and information in evaluation of bioenergy healing methods in routine clinical conditions. These studies may have or have not control group. In this design, a question should exists first and then by considering details such as conditions and duration of intervention, type of patients, number of patients and treatment method observe and evaluate the results. These designs have a great generalization potential, but this design has some limitations concerning the occurrence of bias in patient selection and other conditions.

Research Method

Following the literature review and presentation of appropriate hypothesis and selection of a study design, one should carry out the experiment and assess hypothesis by considering the standard research method. Nield-Anderson and Ameling (2000) have suggested the three following conditions for bioenergy healing studies:

a)   Randomization of sample size.
b)   Having the control group or placebo double-blindness.
c)   Control or placebo.

a)   Randomization and Sample Size

As the sample size of most studies is great, so the researchers measure or apply the research hypothesis on a portion of the population. These selected members are called sample, which is a subpopulation of the whole population and is representative of it. Being representative means there is almost complete similarity between the characteristics of members of sample and the whole population. To achieve this, sample selection should be done randomly, i.e., the equal possibility for each member of the population.

Nield-Anderson and Ameling believe (2000) that most of the studies were carried out by non-patient population and nonrepresentative (volunteer) samples. This decreases the possibility of generalization of results.

b)   Double-Blindness (Blind Assessment)

To prevent any intentional or unintentional bias in the study, in this method the human intervening factors kept unaware of the research process. Following this rule in bioenergy healing, except for distance methods, is so complex.

Ernst and Resch (1995) indicated that designing and maintaining a placebo condition in double-blind studies may be challenging because studies may not remain doubly or even singly blind. Accordingly, we need to continue to monitor the blindedness status among our subjects in our forthcoming study.

Moreover, an interesting rule in sham techniques is that duration and frequency of placebo effect mimics doze dependency of specific effect.

c) Control or Placebo

To confirm the effect of intervention, in most standard studies, control group is used. The control group is usually the same as the case group in different aspects except for the intervening factors that they do not receive it. Following this issue in research provides the possibility of comparison of effectiveness of intervention and elimination of suggesting elements. Bioenergy healing studies require one or more control groups, depending on the research goals. The ways for a neutral intervention in bioenergy-based therapies are applying energy induction by a non-healer person or beyond the electromagnetic nonconductors, without knowledge of the clients.

Quitkin and colleagues (1991) conducted extensive studies on placebo response with regard to function of "time" in subjects with major depression. Their findings indicated that placebo-controlled studies should be long enough to account for that difference in time-effect. Finally, Straus and Cavanaugh (1996) noted that "dose" response effects have also been demonstrated; for example, two placebo capsules were shown to have more pronounced effects than one.

It is an interesting rule in sham techniques that duration and frequency of placebo effect is in accordance with doze dependency of specific effect.

Some of the researchers consider the addition of a placebo arm to their design as the only way to rule out the nonspecific effects of a hands-on/off treatment. Scholars, who are concerned about the chances of their study subjects suspecting the sham treatment, could test their standardization procedures as was done in some studies, and could continue to monitor the status of their subjects, blindedness throughout the study as suggested by authorities in the field of placebo testing (Mansour, Beuche, Laing, Leis & Nurse 1999).

Another problem of clinical studies in holistic medicine is the simultaneous reception of biomedicine intervention (for example in cancer patients). And the elimination of the medical intervention in most of the clinical conditions is not ethically possible. Therefore, results of such studies only indicate the combination of both methods.

Clinical Assessment

As we know, in bioenergy healing, the intervening factor in procedures and remedies are healer and healee as a whole person. Moreover, the factor which undergoes intervention is the healeer as a whole person and not the disease. In addition, it's better to say that these two factors are both affected by healing presence as a transpersonal experiment. On this ground, if we want to summarize bioenergy economy in one sentence, it is "whole heals whole."

This motto demonstrates a top-to-bottom control and also repudiates the linear relationship of subject-object in the clinical atmosphere. Furthermore, it is indicative of the holistic approach of bioenergy economy and shows that the origin of healing is "being" and not "doing." Regarding what was mentioned above, common clinical evaluations cannot be so effective in this approach. What is important in clinical research and work is the measurement of controllable and mutable factors that can affect the healing process. McDonough-Means and colleagues (2004) in their study, "fostering a healing presence and investigating its mediators," introduced the following methodological framework for clinical evaluation of intra/inter/transpersonal factors.

The framework for assessment of nonlocal/nonphysical forces (belief systems and psychospiritual attributes) of those within the healing environment—the healer, the healee, and others within the healing environment (including the experimenter)—may then be constructed. Factors to consider include as follows:

1. Relationships between the persons under study within the system determine the prioritization of the measures taken and administered to persons. For example:

   - The use of prayer (or other related distant healing intervention) by a child's mother may have a more potent effect on the healing of that child than the use of prayer by the nurses caring for the child.
   - The use of a nonconventional energy healing therapy may be unfamiliar to or outside the worldview of some and thereby influence expectancy. This may suggest measurement of

openness, the personality factor most associated with the willingness to try nonconventional therapies, and absorption in the healee or those who are influential within the healee's system.

- When healees and healers are both physically present, assessment of empathy and charisma may be more germane than spirituality and parapsychological attributes when healing is administered from a distance.
- It is important that those who are operative within like levels in relationship to the healee be assessed along similar dimensions and with identical scaling methods to allow for comparisons.

2. Whole-system change is important if healees are being studied over time. For example, belief in the efficacy of a particular healing intervention by those in the environment may shift dramatically throughout the period of a study, and thus exert a differential effect upon the outcome measures via expectancies. Obtaining pre-post length-of-study measures of belief systems from those in the healing environment would be helpful.

McDonough-Means and colleagues expanded their framework to the following issues:

Attitudes, general: Worldview or disposition and psychospiritual traits and states toward the specific (or related) intervention being studied.

Attitudes, specific: Toward both the therapeutic intervention being studied and standard of care (SOC) or control for the condition being treated/studied. *Prior experience:* With SOC and specific (or related) therapeutic intervention being studied with the condition being treated/studied.

Belief in efficacy, general: Of SOC or control and the therapeutic intervention; relative efficacy of therapy ($E_{TX} - E_{cx}$) as % = $E_{Tx}/E_{TX} + E_{Cx}$.

Belief in efficacy, specific: As above, but to each subject's condition, paired with assessment of illness severity; global belief in efficacy (EG), improvement regardless of treatment (may reflect rater's optimism) specific to each subject may be embedded within ETX; thus expectancy $E=E_{TX} - E_G$.

Assessment of benefit: Perceived clinical progress of the condition being studied and the whole—person at the end of the study and attribution of cause and risks. If raters are blinded to group assignment, obtain rater's group assignment guess with confidence rating, to assess bias of this rating.

Many diagnostic indices such as visual analogue scales (VAS) and functional assessment of chronic illness therapy (FACIT) were employed to assess the general state of the individual and the general trend of treatment, which are analogical but clinically effective.

The 100-mm visual analogue scale (VAS) has been widely used and is suitable for capturing subjective ratings. In the ensuing study, energy healers were asked to choose the scaling method for their clinical assessment of the subject and for rating energy field descriptors. They chose the 100 mm VAS over a Likert or numeric analog scale as more compatible with their "altered state" (i.e., meditative, intuitive, and simultaneous versus linear and quantitative). For similar reasons, the wording of questions was changed from "How ill is . . . now" and "How much stress does . . . have now" to "What is your overall sense of . . . illness now" and "What is your overall sense of . . . response to stress now." Questions that provide more holistic and positive ratings of subjects are desirable (e.g., how "well" versus how "ill" is . . . or a rating of "overall" sense of wellbeing over . . . [time period]).

When the focus of research outcomes of healing presence is the healee as a whole person, the reliance on disease-specific or organ-specific outcome measures constitutes a valuable but incomplete assessment. The healer and the treatment may catalyze a continuum of changes that are multifactorial and multidimensional and often subtle and cumulative or progressive. Measurement of multivariate, global outcomes with appropriate statistical-analytic tools becomes necessary. Multidimensional scales such as the functional assessment of chronic illness therapy (FACIT), which can assess biopsychosociospiritual status in a coordinated set of modules, may be useful. There is the reason is that extensive rating scales of health and well-being can capture the integrated overall outcomes that separate dimension-specific questionnaires may miss.

Measurement of the degree of positive well-being, in addition to the reduction of negative conditions (e.g., diseases), is possible with some available instruments for mood and positive states of mind. This may also be reflected by traditional measures such as disease incidence and complications, medications, utilization of health-care resources including length of hospitalization, growth, and participation in ordinary life functions. These data, although broad, are regarded as acting as interactive variables and avoid the bias of premature focus upon predetermined, more focused outcomes: "The key is not found under the lamp simply because that is where the light is" (Donough-Means, Kreitzer & Bell 2004).

Quality of life can be accommodated as a multidimensional outcome measure that has been used widely in recent years. One of the measurements of this index is WHO QOL (quality of life), which evaluates QOL in six axes and by twenty-four items.

The six axes are:

I. Pain as discomfort
II. Psychological state
III. Level of independence
IV. Social relationships
V. Environment
VI. Spirituality/Religion/Personal beliefs

Each WHOQOL facet can be identified as a description of a behavior, a state of being, a capacity or potential or a subjective perception or experience. For example, pain is a subjective perception or experience; fatigue may be defined as a state; mobility may be defined either as a capacity (ability to move around) or as a behavior (actual report of walking). A definition was written for each of the facets of quality of life covered by the WHOQOL assessment (WHO, 1998). Moreover, direct observation or video records of behaviors (Caudell 1996) as well as measurement of physiological variable of biomarkers can be used for behavioral assessment of client in treatment. However, owing to the high cost and stress of these methods, it is better to use them just when necessary.

Research Dilemmas

A short review of reliable studies carried out on bioenergy healing demonstrates a range of studies extending from in vitro studies to clinical trials, qualitative studies, and case reports. A psychological analysis of these studies indicates that:

1. Precise and quantitative studies neglect many aspects of healer—healee relationship.
2. Qualitative studies that are more congruent with the real circumstances of healing are of a lower precision and generalization potentiality.
3. In vitro studies, distant healings have the lowest bias and obviously reveal the physical and qidynamic bioenergy effects.
4. Hitherto, there has been no precise and clear semiology for interpretation of the data collected from various apparatus for bioenergy measurement. Therefore, standardization of the independent variable "bioenergy" and generalization of these interventions is not feasible. Standard quantitative studies can only be considered of analogical value because each individual, intention, and attunement owns a unique and specific bioenergy formula, which is in interaction with space-time and other individuals, as well.
5. Putativeness of bioenergy and ungeneralizability of the healing experience is not indicative of invalidity of this field of knowledge. On the other hand, it demonstrates the organic and dynamic nature of research and the structural deficiency of quantitative studies in reflecting profoundly relational experience of healing.
6. It seems that major parts of these methodological problems will not be resolved by advancement of science as it relates to the fundamental uncertainty of this area of physics and biosemiotics. However, it should be noted that if we want to consider

physician—patient relationship and psychosocial factors of the patient in biomedicine, we will be best with the same problem in generalization and certainty.

7. To arrange bioenergy healing protocols, analogical quantitative studies and qualitative studies are both required. Quantitative studies provide the possibility to understand the processes analytically, while qualitative studies provide the chance to comprehend the healing conditions paternalistically.

As it can be inferred from the above-mentioned research considerations, by employing a complex thinking pattern, we can comprehend the healing presence correctly. Linear and reductionistic thinking will only provide a blurred and opaque purview to this field. Considering the local and nonlocal effects of bioenergy not only can reveal the role of intentional bias, but also demonstrate how the attitude and intention of the researcher can affect the results of the study. A case in point is the Hawthorne effect where human beings change when they are "watched" (Roethlisberger & Dickson 1939).

There is current, incremental evidence that putting certain healing phenomena into an experimental context (i.e., creating a closed system for observation) may in itself alter the process (Rosenthal 1994; Walach, Schmidt, Dirhold & Nosch 2002). This appears to be especially true for a phenomenon such as healing presence, in which not only local, but also nonlocal or transcendental mediators may play a role, to the extent even that the beliefs of the experimenters could influence study outcomes (Donough-Means, Kreitzer & Bell 2004).

In parapsychology, Schlitz and Wiseman have shown that the same remote viewing protocol bears in positive evidence for nonlocal effects, when implemented by a believer in psychic phenomena. However, the same protocol may breed negative evidence for such effects when implemented by a skeptic (Schlitz & Haight 1984; Wiseman & Schlitz 1997). The experimenters' impact on tested variables not only can be effected directly, but also through the influence which it exerts on the higher and lower order levels of the organization. The impact of experimenter behavior and belief on the outcome of the study merits due consideration, which in its own turn entails assessment of these potentially relevant factors in studies of healing presence (Donough-Means, Kreitzer & Bell 2004).

Surrounding physical environment, lower levels of system organization at the level of physical-chemical and the toxic and esthetic (Bronzaft 2002; Jasnoski 1992), artificial and natural (Gross et al. 1998; Simson & Straus 1998), and characteristics of the sensory environment, all merit evaluation with regard to their impact on healing presence. Human beings may maintain an "ecological unconsciousness" that when exposed to natural surroundings is stirred and stimulated and fosters benefits for physical and mental health (Thoms 2003). Improved recovery from surgery (Ulrich 1984), stress (Hartig et al. 2003), enhanced attention (Laumann, Carling & Stormark 2003), and decreased distractibility and enhanced inner calm (Korpela, Klemettila & Hietanen 2002) have all been demonstrated with exposure to natural settings. If subtle energetic interactions contribute to healing, then careful assessment of the background electromagnetic environment during a study is also essential (Hintz et al. 2003).

Concerning all these intrinsic and extrinsic factors and interventions each study make in bioenergy healing reflection indicates that to take the advantage of these effective clinical methods, we should pursue bioenergy economy principles in research. Moreover, instead of emphasizing the precision of or similarity with the complex and vague clinical conditions, we should strive a balanced and multidimensional method for the study of this deeply-dynamic and communicative phenomenon. As it was mentioned, various research methodologies should be employed to explain different aspects of bioenergy healing.

Appendix A

Reiki: A Brief, Traditional Healing System

Reiki is a simplified Eastern bioenergy discipline. The simplicity and facility in education and employment make it one of the most popular self-healing techniques. Reiki is a method of transferring universal life-giving energy for the harmony of the body, mind, and soul. It addresses both the cause and effect of illness. It is transferred by gently placing the hands on your own body or that of another person. No religious philosophy is necessary to do Reiki, although it is thought of as a spiritual system. People of varying philosophical views, ages, and life circumstances can practice this loving art (Hall 2000).

Reiki Principles

After years of study, research, and practical experiences in medicine, psychology, mysticism, religions, and healing methods such as *Qigong*, Kundalini Yoga, and also getting familiar with the health system during the time served as the vice chancellor of Japanese ministry of health, Mikao Usui (1865-1926) founded the Reiki (Lubek, 1991; Hurwitz, 2001).

Usui did not found Reiki on complex and hard exercises of internal energy release, but it was based on openness and coordination with universal energy field. The coordination of *Rei* and *Ki* are easily achieved by being in accordance with the master. In this regard, induction of energy-information system gives the individual a higher level of coordination in the energetic and emotional system (Goli, 2008).

Usui, the founder of Reiki, in his first healing experiments, understood the necessity of considering the spiritual and psychological intervention, along with the energetic ones. So he proposed very simple lifestyle modification principles for those who were healed.

By considering the psychological and spiritual aspects, Usui established the five Reikis' principles, which moderate the individual's lifestyle, and in spite of its simplicity, properly can guide the health-oriented behaviors of the individual.

The principles of Reiki and their cognitive and behavioral aspects are briefly described in the following:

First Principle: Just for Today, Do Not Worry

The keywords of this principle are "just for today" and "worry" that are explained below.

"Just for Today": This is an emphasis on the basic humanistic psychology of "now and here." Antecedent psychologists, by focusing on the past, concern the personality as the result of nonconscious suppressed elements (psychoanalytical term) or learned habits (behaviorism term) during childhood. Psychologists soon understood that these approaches are not consistent with behavioral and human characteristics and people are not, as psychoanalysts and behaviorist mentioned, captivated by their past. Regarding this, humanistic approaches, by focusing on present experiences, made popular more simple therapeutic method with higher level of cost-benefit.

The pioneer of gestalt therapy, Perls, believed that the reason of not being in present time is uncompleted gestalts which its solution is to play responsible role at present time (Shultz & Shultz 2004).

By emphasizing "today," Usui has a psychologic view over the issue and mentions living in the present moment, being here, and attendance as the key elements of health in this lifestyle.

Some psychologists believe that worry is a cognitive subsystem, interacts with behavioral, emotional, and physical subsystems, and is the basis of anxiety disorders (Borkovec & Newman 1999).

Worry is the cognitive and basic component of anxiety and relates to expecting to encounter with vague threatening factor in future and also testing oneself in this confrontation. Worry generally has an attention bias toward unpleasant stimulations. If one concentrates on "just today," mind automatically will not be diverted toward future and probable negative events. By leading the attention toward today, this blocks the activated cognitive route of anxiety.

Concerning the energetic and spiritual aspect, the Reiki energy flow of one is activated by thinking and meditating over this principle (Fis, 1998).

Second Principle: Just for Today, Do Not Get Angry

Anger, besides enjoyment and happiness, compose the main human effects. By presenting the second principle, Usui explains the key to control and keep all intense emotions. In the first principle, tempting emotions such as worry are important while in the second principle rough, impulsive, comprehensive, and stimulating emotions are of great importance.

Usui suggests moving softly toward the unconditional love (ibid), since anger is one of the biggest communicative disorders and obstructs the flow of kindness that is the basis for relation of human with himself, others, and the universe.

In this regard, this approach leads the individual from the impulsive emotions to permanent emotions that are in accordance with the organism tendency.

Once again, emphasizing today, places the mind "here and now." Also by defining a time interval, a big task is divided into several smaller tasks with higher chance for success. In this way, by achieving one-day successes in affection control and gaining skills and self-confidence, the individual can gradually alters his adaptation model and personality.

Third Principle: Honor Your Parents, Teachers, and Elders

McKenzie (1998) interprets this principle in this way: Respect those who taught us life and knowledge and appreciate them.

But Fis (1998) believes that Usui had some meaning beyond this, as "the teacher is within yourself."

It seems that this explanation is based on the fact that parents, teachers, and elders are the symbols of our psych roots. In this regard, many psychoanalysts know psychoanalysis as the reconstruction of parent—child relationship. The parents are not only father and mother, but also all those who played a parental role in our life. Respecting the parents is respecting the roots and depth of our own life.

Relationship with parents, teachers, and elderly accompanied by respect and appreciation not only reduces the internal and external conflicts, but also is a way of preventing and treating the pervasive modern world disease of alienation and unrootedness.

On the other hand, respecting the elderly is respecting the life, admiring the parents is appreciating yourself and respecting the teachers is appreciation of knowledge and wisdom. All these appreciations are giving the meaning to life.

Fourth Principle: Earn Your Living Honestly

This principle develops sense of responsibility (McKenzic 1998). As it is mentioned in Reiki background, when Usui proposed these principles, he lived with beggars and thieves and there he understood the importance of lifestyle and its changes to achieve the remedy and total health.

Recommending the moral principle of earn livelihood in this method of healing, demonstrates the Usui's attention to the effect of social and spiritual factors on health.

Focusing this principle can improve the direct, active, and responsible understanding of life. This principle focuses on honest earning of life (Fis, 1998), as life is something obtainable, not passive and textual. It is an aim, which should be achieved actively.

Fifth Principle: Show Gratitude to Everything

According to Fis (1998), previously mentioned principles leads us to this principle as all things exist within ourselves. Just we should allow this knowledge to flow into our consciousness. He believes that the individual who shows gratitude toward all living organisms and things lives in silence and internal and external peace.

McKenzie (1998) says that this principle fortifies the blessed feeling. Positive emotional relation with universe separates the individual from his conditional alienation and puts him into the context of universe. In this way, the individual experiences comprehensive coordination with universe. This attitude brings us higher psychological, neurologic, communicative, and immunological coordination and makes higher level of health achievable for us.

To put it into nutshell, the first two principles are to lead the individual to the experience of here and now and to relief him from the reaction emotions toward future, past, and others. The third principle is coordinating with our symbolic spirit roots and giving value to life and knowledge. The fourth principle helps us to achieve a direct understanding of life and participate in it actively and with sense of responsibility. Finally, the fifth principle denotes the coordination with all elements of the universe.

Thinking, meditation, and following these principles can provide the conditions of lifestyle and personality modification.

Basic Concepts of Reiki

Reiki consists of two Japanese words: "Rei" means, the superior power or the divine wisdom, and "Ki" means, the life-giving energy (Rand 2000). Stein (2000) describes "Ki" as energy, air, breath, wind, vital breath, essence of life, and finally the activating energy of universe.

Rand (2000) believes that Reiki that consists of two Japanese words should be translated into English carefully, as words in Japanese have different levels of meaning. So the context of the word should also be taken into consideration. As these two words are used in the context of spiritual healing, their translation should not be limited to daily conversational meanings. For instance, in dictionaries, "Rei" is usually translated into spirit and ghost, and "Ki" as vapor or fog. If these words be translated in this manner, then their meaning would be limited.

In a spiritual structure, "Rei" can be defined as the superior consciousness that leads to creation and universe performance. "Rei" is a subtle wisdom that penetrates in everything, either living or nonliving. At the human level, "Rei" is accessible to help us when necessary and acts as a guidance source in our life.

"Ki" is the nonphysical energy, which gives life to everything. "Ki" flows in everything such as plants, animals, and human. When the "Ki" level of somebody is high, he has the feeling of power, competency, and preparedness for joyful life and vice versa. Reiki practitioners believe that we obtain the "Ki" from breath, food, sunshine, and sleep (ibid).

The combination of "Rei" and "Ki" makes the word "Reiki." According to aforementioned information, Reiki means "the spiritual, guided bioenergy" (see Whelan & Wishnia 2003). This is a competent definition of this healing method.

Stein (2000) believes Reiki as a Kundalini discipline. These systems are based on the supposition of the possibility of modification of Prana-vayu, chakras, and the brain. In Sanskrit, "vayu" means air, and when used in combination with "prana," it defines the personal vital power (Gopikrishna 1998). This description only distinguishes the "Ki" dimension of "Reiki," and ontologic and cosmologic aspects are not defined.

Considering this, Reiki is an bioenergetic intervention to coordinate biofield with the universal energy field.

Attunement Concept

Each individual has vital force and healing ability (Neild-Anderson & Ameling 2000), and relates with his environment and other people as a dynamic and unique field of energy (Rogers 1970) according to Martha Rogers's openness theory, human and his surrounding environment are in continuous, permanent energy exchange (ibid). However, employing this power and potential and opening the doors of this interaction with environment happens through the attenuation mechanism.

The process of transferring bioenergy from teacher to student is called attunement. This is an bioenergy transfer process and the role of the teacher is to facilitate the process (Neild-Anderson & Ameling 2000).

During the attunement process, the teacher of Reiki use mantra and symbols to crate and strengthen the health vibrations to increase the individual's capability of meridianing and receiving bioenergy. Attunements are systems to activate and increase the meridianing ability of the receiver. In this way, the life power automatically flows through the body and spirit of the individual (ibid). Regarding the aforementioned integrative health model (physical, psychological, energetic, and spiritual), the attunement, an energetic process, is affected by psychological, physical, and spiritual factors. So, the effects of attunement are different in various people. The reverse is also correct, i.e., the energetic attunement process affects the individual's physical, psychological, and spiritual aspects. These phenomena and how they occur will be explained in the chapter of mechanisms.

Reiki Symbols

One of the most important Reiki conceptualizations is in the form of symbols. The five symbols that are widely used in Reiki and are usually presented and employed in levels two and three are as follows:

Cho-ku-rei
Sei-he-ki
Hon-sha-ze-nen
Dai-Ko-Myo
Raku

These symbols, which root in the traditional Tibetan tantric mysticism, are considered as the transformers that shape the bioenergy and are employed for psyche purification and therapeutic purposes (see, e.g., figure A 1.1).

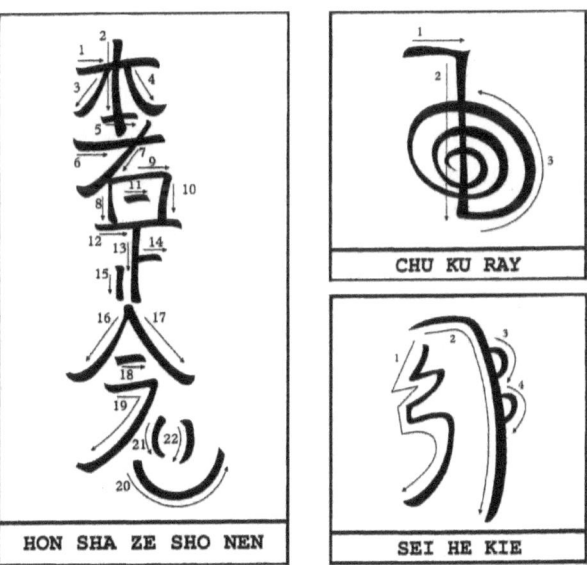

Figure A 1.1. The main psychospiritual symbols of Reiki, which are drawn as showed in diagrams.

Cho-ku-rei is used to empower and amplify the *Rei* flow, while *Sei-he-ki* is to maintain the relation of earth and heaven, top and down, human and divinity, and generally to organize and release excitement via unification of human and universe. *Hon-sha-ze-nen* is usually used to transfer the healing power of Reiki in time and place. So it is used for distance healing and purification of archetypes (Stein 2000).

Reiki users believe that symbols induce the mentioned effects in a meaningful and obvious way. Is this an induced effect? Or symbols are in fact, the archetypes of our collective unconscious that are decoded in our unconscious and cause these changes?

Is it possible that these effects or even the symbols are not transferred to receiver by direct induction, but indirectly, through extrasensory perception (ESP)?

Some Reiki teachers have reported that even prior to presentation of symbols, just after the primary attunement, some images were produced in mind of some users; they understood these were Reiki symbols, later (ibid).

Reiki symbols can be considered as controlled symbolic visualization, since it is used as superficial manner. On the other hand, when it focuses on meditation upon and contemplation of spiritual aspects of symbols, it can be considered as symbolization toward psychospiritual evolution.

Anyhow, there are several reports on spontaneous imagination of various symbolic images other than formal Reiki symbols by users that are not treated systematically.

Meditative contemplation upon the fivefold principles of Reiki is regarded as subsystems of psychospiritual evolution and obviously is employed to actualize these principles in personality and life of the individual.

Educational Principles of Reiki

Ever-increasing inclination of people to complementary and alternative medicine (CAM) in recent decades resulted in quantitative and qualitative changes of health problems, some scientific achievements, and some cultural and spiritual issues. This has made new challenges for health systems. A short look at the history demonstrate that people usually understand social and health changes sooner than scientific and executive organizations, and the role of these organizations is just to organize and explain these currents and not creating them. The present gap between needs and requirements of the societies and current health and therapeutic services has led to managerial disharmony, unprofessional and unscientific attitudes, dangerous interventions in treatment process, and relative lack of confidence in formal health service systems. Thus, many countries have passed new laws and organized new research, treatment, and education programs in this field (e.g., Fisher & Ward 1994, WHO 2001, WHCCAMP 2001). Teaching of complementary and alternative medicine to medical disciplines in fellowship courses and academic certifications in medical courses has been performed in developed countries in recent years (Weeks 2001). Various studies are indicative of academic acceptance of these CAM educational programs (e.g., Wetzed, Eisenberg & Kaptchuk 1994).

However, transformation of clinical medicine from an exclusive experimental paradigm to an ethnosocial paradigm, based on experimental findings, has provided the opportunity for development of these treatments (Goli & Zamani 2004).

Concerning the ever-increasing growth of these services and people's inclination to these therapeutic methods, some experts suggest the following strategies to cover these needs and development of the knowledge and skills of the trainees:

1) Holding in-service training courses.
2) Holding educational seminars.
3) Holding journal clubs and case-report sessions.
4) Carrying out clinical trials.
5) Methodological development of scientific communities.
6) Supporting research institutes.
7) Founding research and information centers in medical science universities.
8) Translation and compilation of scientific textbooks.
9) Understanding health beliefs, attitudes, and behaviors in people.
10) Scientific and executive organization of traditional practitioners (Farzanegan 2002).

A Short Look at the Reiki Levels

Contrary to many complementary and alternative methods, Reiki is so simple and does not require long training (Nield-Anderson & Ameling 2000).

During the attunement process, the master transfers Reiki to the trainee. Mantras and symbols are used to activate the trainee capability for openness to the universe life-giving energy (Whelan & Wishnia 2003).

Now, Reiki is presented in three levels traditionally (Nield-Anderson & Ameling 2000). Generally, at the first level, the trainee gets acquainted with the Reiki background. The trainee at this level receives attunement.

Reiki trainee at this level is only allowed to work on himself, his/her family, and friends. The trainee at the second level gets familiar with healing system and receives attunement of this level (ibid). They are allowed to deal with patients. Finally, at the third level, trainees will reach master level and can teach others.

In traditional method of Reiki teaching, each level is defined and implemented in a rigid and inflexible manner, and no psychological and behavioral skill is taught. In this method, no explanation is given about the manner and mechanism of Reiki and energy currents, and psychological and spiritual guides are not offered to the trainees.

Usui education system, which is implemented only in his institute, is based on six levels (six to one). This is in contrast with the modern levels of one to three or four. It is interesting to note that Usui considered himself to be at the second level but had kept the way open to higher levels than him. He never used the term *master* for Reiki trainees and even himself and the terms *master* and *grand master* were introduced by Ms. Takata and other Western teachers. The first four levels are called *Shoden* or primary levels (six to three). The fifth level is called Okuden or internal training, which consists of *Okuden Zenki* (the first half) and *Okuden Kuki* (the second half). The master level is called *Shinpiden* or symbolic training (Lubeck 1991).

In Usui traditional approach, Ki exercises and using *Hui Yin* position (contraction of perineum) does not exist, and there are no alternative symbols to teach symbols, and anything except traditional Reiki issues are considered "not Reiki."

Stein (2000) regarded nontraditional and more comprehensive methods for training of Reiki trainees more suitable. He believed that more comprehensive information and more introduced training choices enhance the motivation of the trainee for learning and then transferring it. Concentrating on the integrative health model (see ch. II) reveals the importance of psychological and physical systems along with energetic and spiritual systems. Recognizing personality and psychological aspects in the framework of needs, conflicts, abnormal behaviors, and methods of confrontation and management to control them is the first step in the teaching of Reiki.

Stein (2000) considered this training step to include identification and analysis of needs and limitations of the trainee and then managing them, because each person has a specific psychological structure that can be presented in his intervention method.

This psychological analysis was founded by Freud. He believed that before performing therapeutic intervention and analysis of others personality, the psychoanalyst should become aware of the suppressed materials in his own unconsciousness to avoid transferring them to his/her client via projection mechanism. These projects can have cognitive and behavioral aspects as well as bioenergetic aspects, and energetic disorders of the practitioner can influence the client (Goli 2008).

Paying attention to this issue is important in behavioral and cognitive approaches as the psychoanalyst may be considered standard and clients may assimilate him/her. For instance, the relaxed status of the therapist is as important as the training of relaxation (ibid).

Considering these factors in Reiki training system can be complementary to energetic and spiritual interventions and increases the depth of the effects.

Therefore, it is recommended that the Reiki trainee learn the Reiki for him/her to have enough time and chance to be prepared for the therapeutic atmosphere. To achieve this, it is better to give him/herself daily Reiki after learning Reiki I in order to become skilled in management and guidance of energy. Then, after few weeks, he/she can give others Reiki.

At first, the trainee is better not to consider Reiki II and III and after becoming fluent in Reiki I, begins Reiki II. Similarly, one can move from direct Reiki (contact or noncontact touch therapy) to distance Reiki.

Getting familiar with the mechanism of these methods can be useful (Stein 2000).

Two items should be considered in memorization of symbols according to traditional methods:

To draw the lines and then the direction of vectors in their drawing, symbols should be sent for healing to the client first and then imagine them by drawing.

After this step, Ki exercises begin for at least a few weeks, thirty minutes for each session. These exercises are useful for deep-energy experience. Some believe that it is better to begin these exercises with *Hui Yin* position—contraction of anal and perineal muscles—and gradually increase its duration (ibid). Nevertheless, many therapists believe that this is not essential or even effective (Hurwitz 2001).

Continuing these exercises, one should feel the flow of Ki in the body and then the ability to change this feeling will be achieved. When these states occur fluently, then Reiki III can be started.

It is better to begin Reiki III with Dai-Ko-Myo symbols and avoid non-Reiki and personal symbols at this stage. *Dai-Ko-Myo* symbols are used for direct and distance healing. When the trainee becomes familiar with direct healing, five main symbols of Reiki and Ki exercise, it is the time to begin Reiki III (Stein 2000).

After learning attunement, it should be practiced at any possible time until the trainee become fluent in it. In Reiki team training, exercises and healing action can be done simultaneously.

When all exercises were done fluently and the attunement process was performed, Reiki training can be started. Before the class, it is better to give Reiki I to a person which can be a member of the family. Then, the process will be repeated for other persons in groups of less than five members. When the individual's capacity for attunement enhanced, he can work with larger groups (Stein 2000).

Regarding the existence of suggesting and non-suggesting elements in Reiki process, the Reiki education place is better to be a convenient, simple place and based on the teacher's view be formal or informal. Classes with rows of chairs are not suitable for this purpose. If there are chairs, during the healing process it is better to take the chairs out of the class or arrange them around the class in a circular manner.

Maintaining the Hui Yin position during the attunement process is difficult for the receiving person and as it was mentioned it is not necessary.

Methods of teaching Reiki to children need consideration. For this purpose, it is better to invite children that are able to keep the time of the class. Presence of the mother or one of the family members makes the child to do what he/she perform and the accompanying person will learn the way she/he can help the child. Children usually learn Reiki positions but cannot spend much time on each of them.

As it was mentioned before, there are three levels of Reiki training (Nield-Anderson & Ameling 2000) and in a formal view each level contain an specific structure and educational program. Different methods can be employed for better education in a way that trainees learn what is more effective for them (ibid).

Appendix B

Yoga: A Comprehensive, Traditional Healing System

Opposing to the Reiki's to-the-point and simple bioenergy approach to vital force, yoga's orthodox discipline is comprehensive, complex, and very long term.

Yoga is a magnificent psychological, philosophical, and lifestyle tradition and several contemporary schools of psychology and philosophy directly or indirectly have been inspired of.

According to *patan jali's yoga sutras*, the main reference of yoga, this is introduced asa nonreligious, practical way to salvation and unity with universe.

Yoga $\sqrt{yuj}$ means integration or wholeness. The yogic concept of the working of the body and mind is that there is, in both, a homoeostatic mechanism which contributes to balanced, integrating functioning, and that each person has an inherent power of adaptation and consciousness evolution. Yoga considers the human being as a whole and does not divide human condition into body, mind, and spirit and even human and nature.

Four basic approach to wholeness and unity exist in Yogic tradition which complement each other: *Raja Yoga* (the path of observing and controlling of mind-body activities), *Jnana Yoga* (the path of esoteric knowledge), *Bahkti Yoga* (the path of devotion to the supreme consciousness) and *Karma Yoga* (the path of work for work's sake) (see Vivekananda, 2007a; 2006; 2001; 2007b).

All of these disciplines are various *Prana* equations for the sake of consciousness evolution and coordinating of body's mind, soul, and spirit.

Raja Yoga is the most common and systematic discipline of yoga tradition. *Patanjali* enumerated eight principal limbs of yogic practice as follows:

1. Moral restraint (*Yama*): gentleness, truthfulness, honesty, chastity, and generosity (social code)
2. Discipline (*Niyama*): purity, contentment, asceticism, study, and devotion (observances)
3. Postures and movements (*asana*)
4. Breathings (*pranayama*)
5. Withdrawal of the senses (*pratyahara*)
6. Concentration (*dharana*)
7. Meditation (*dhyana*)
8. Super consciousness (*samadhi*)

These techniques are employed in liberation, absorption, and conducting of bioenergy (*prana*).

But *prana* denotes "life force" or "bioenergy." It is also the medium through with matter and mind are linked to consciousness (Micozzi & Singh, 2006)

The spinal cord, with the reproductive equipment at one end and the ventricular cavity in 'the brain at the other, is the largest repository of the life force, or prana, in the human body. This life force is a biochemical substance of a most complex formation, extremely subtle and volatile, having its roots probably in the subatomic levels of matter. Belief in the efficacy of yoga as a time-honored method of self-realization ipso facto means belief in prang, for the whole science of yoga is built on the possibility of employing prana as an instrument for effecting a metamorphosis of the brain and raising it to higher levels of perception. In every form of yoga, with a meditative technique or discipline of the breath, the first object intended to be influenced is prana (Krishna, 1998).

Gopikrishna (1996) explains the vibrational worldview of yoga as follow:

"In order to obtain a clearer idea of how the forces of life and the Law of Evolution can be conceived of, in the context of the current theories about the elementary forces of matter, it is sufficient to say that the classical concepts of extremely minute solid objects which combined, like diminutive bricks, to form molecules and compounds has been demolished. The material world has now to be imagined as a stupendous ocean of wave-like patterns of probable interconnections of which it is not possible to forma precise image by any means possible to man.

"A material particle, such as an electron," says Hermann Weyl, "is merely a small domain of the electric field, within which the field strength assumes enormously high values, indicating that comparatively huge field energy is concentrated in a very small space. Such an energy knot, which by no means is clearly delineated against the remaining field, propagates through empty space, like a water wave across the surface of a lake; there is no such thing as one and the same substance of which the electron consists at all times."

From this plain description of the invisible levels of matter, we can readily form the image of a human being, as he actually exists, as a fluidal field of interconnected and interacting forces devoid of the form, shape, size, color ti i id substance, presented to our mind by the senses and their brain. With this picture, the world of name and form vanishes away completely. This dissolution of the objective world into Consciousness is a phenomenon known to Yogis for thousands of years. Universal Consciousness (Brahman) with its "Maya-Shakti" existing behind the energy field of the universe, lies completely beyond the range of our observation, the real source of all creation, yet entirely all of and unaffected by its constant movement and activity. The Law of Evolution springing from the "Maya-Shakfi" of the Creator is operative in the finest levels of our organic structures, subtler than the neurons and their constituents or, in other words, in the invisible energy fields to which they owe their existence, shape, and form. The issue has been touched in passing to bring out colossal implications of the law of yoga, as a discipline designed to remodel the human brain at its deepest levels completely hidden from our knowledge and sight."

Yogic Interventions and Bioenergetic Equations

Yoga is a consciousness evolution knowledge, which controls lifestyle modalities via:

o   Physical awareness in *Hath yoga* (physical activity, Breathing physical and cleansing)
o   Mindfulness (*Pratyahara, Dharana, Dhiana,* and *Samadhi*)
o   Bioenergetic awareness in *Kondalini Yoga* (awaking the intrinsic energy and connecting to cosmic energy)
o   And so:
o   Chronobiological awareness in *swara yoga* (biorhythms and lifecycle)
o   Moral awareness (*Yama* and *Niyama*) (see Goli, 2003)

Physical Awareness

In continues we only present brief introductions to the psychosomatic modalities and techniques.

Yogic physical trainings include hundreds of postures/movements (*Asanas, Bandhas, Mudras*) and several breathing techniques (*PranaYama*), which are preformed in an aware, gentle, and coordinated manner.

Coordination of movement/posture, breathing, and mental activities is a main key of these techniques. Each of *asanas* of yoga performs in different levels of skillfulness and consciousness from body awareness to body-breathing harmonization and finally bioenergetic awareness. For this purposes, Hatha yoga course is started with simple physical training and body awareness and continued with breathing harmonies (see, e.g., figure B 2.1).

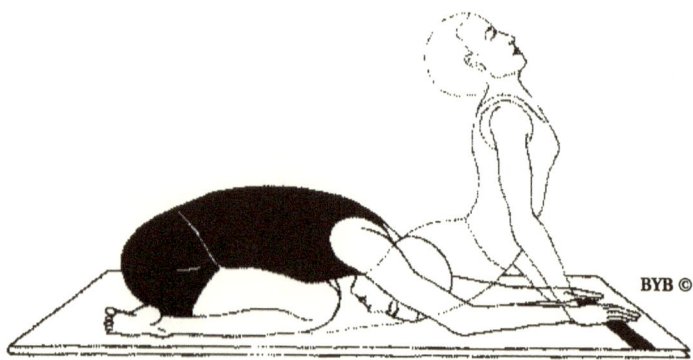

Figure B 2.1. A sample of the asanas and its psychophysical instructions (quoted from Satyananda 1996, 126-127, with kind permission from Satyananda).

Shashank Bhujangasana (striking cobra pose)

Assume marjari-asana, placing the palms flat on the floor beneath the shoulders about half a metre apart.

Move into shashankasana with the arms outstretched in front of the shoulders.

Then, without moving the position of the hands, slowly move the chest forward, sliding it just above the floor until it is in line with the hands.

Move the chest further forward and then upward, as the arms straighten, and lower the pelvis to the floor.

Ideally, the nose and chest should just brush the surface of the floor as the body moves forward like the movement of a snake. Do not strain to achieve this.

Try to bring the hips as near to the floor as possible.

In the final position, the arms should be straight, the back arched and the head raised as in bhujangasana. The navel does not touch the floor.

Hold this position for a few seconds, retaining the breath.

Slowly raise the buttocks and move backwards, keeping the arms straight, returning to shashankasana.

Do not try to reverse the previous movement but keep the arms straight.

This is one round.

Relax the whole body for a short time before starting another round.

Practice 5 to 7 rounds.

Breathing: Inhale on the forward movement.

Hold the breath for a few seconds in the final position.

Exhale while returning to shashankasana.

Awareness: Physical—on synchronising the movement with the breath.

Spiritual—on swadhisthana chakra.

Sequence: This asana may be practiced directly after shashankasana and followed by tadasana.

Benefits: Shashank bhujangasana gives similar benefits to bhujangasana and shashankasana. However, the benefits of the latter postures come from maintaining the final position, whereas shashank bhujangasana acts mainly by alternately flexing the spine backward and forward.

This asana gently tones the female reproductive organs, alleviates menstrual disorders and is an excellent postnatal asana, strengthening and tightening the abdominal and pelvic region. It tones and improves the functioning of the liver, kidneys and other visceral organs. It is particularly useful for relieving back pain and general stiffness of the spine as it helps to stimulate and balance all the spinal nerves.

Practice note: The hand position should not change throughout the entire practice.

Pranayamas are breathing technique for modulating the autonomic nervous function and the flow of *prana* into the vital systems. In a classic yogic program, pranayamas starts after a few month asana training and so some of necessary physical cleansing (see: e.g., figure B 2.2).

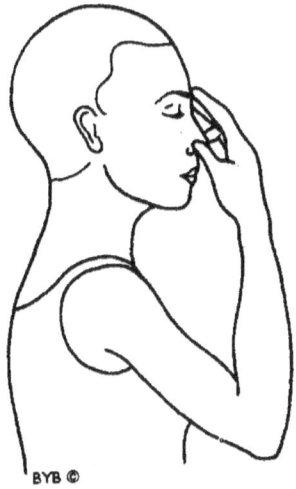

Figure B 2.2. A sample of the Pranayamas and its psychophysical instructions (quoted from Satyananda 1996: 384-385, with kind permission from Satyananda)

Awareness: Physical—on the breath and the counting.

Mental—it is easy for the mind to wander during nadi shodhana. Simply be aware of this wandering tendency of the mind, continue the practice and the count. This will automatically encourage the awareness to return to the practice.

Spiritual—on ajna chakra.

Precautions: Depending on the phase of the moon, one of the two nostrils usually becomes strongly dominant during the time of sunrise and sunset. This is a period of intense *swara*, 'breath', activity and it is not advisable to alter the flows at this time. Under no circumstance should the breath be forced. Never breathe through the mouth. Proceed carefully and only under expert guidance. At the slighter sign of discomfort, reduce the duration of inhalation/exhalation/retention and, if necessary, discontinue the practice for the day. Nadi shodhana should never be rushed.

Sequence: Nadi shodhana should be practiced after asanas and heating or cooling pranayamas, and before bhramari and ujjayi pranayamas. The best time to practice is from 4 to 6 am; however, it may be performed any time during the day except after meals.

Duration: 5 to 10 rounds or 10 to 15 minutes daily.

Benefits: Nadi shodhana ensures that the whole body is nourished by an extra supply of oxygen. Carbon dioxide is efficiently expelled and the blood is purified of toxins. The brain centers are stimulated to work nearer to their optimum capacity. It also induces tranquility, clarity of thought and concentration, and is recommended for those engaged in mental work. It increases vitality and lowers levels of stress and anxiety by harmonizing the pranas. It clears pranic blockages and balances ida and pingala nadis. Causing sushumna nadi to flow, which leads to deep states of meditation and spiritual awakening.

Practice note: Development of nadi shodhana is intended to take place over a long period of time. Each technique should be practiced for a minimum of 6 months, except for technique 1 which may be practiced for 2 to 4 weeks. Developing the ratios and timing of the breath in each technique may even take years.

Techniques 1 and 2 prepare the lungs and the nervous system for techniques 3 and 4 which introduce antar and bahir kumbhaka, internal and external breath retention. Mastery of the later techniques may take some time to realize as the body and mind need to adjust to the effects of extended breath retention. The full benefits of this practice will be obtained by systematically perfecting each level rather than by struggling prematurely with the advanced techniques.

Note: *The word* nadi *means 'Channel' or flow' of energy and* shodhana *means 'Purification'. Nadi shodhana, therefore, means that practice which purifies the nadis. The number 24, used for timing the breath, derives from classical texts which use the Gayatri mantra as a metre to measure the length of pranayamas; the Gayatri mantra is made up of 24 individual mantras.*

Some of yogic breathing technique tranquilize mind and body, some of them arouse, and some establish equilibrium. See incorrect prana yama may cause hiccups, asthma, headache, and other ailments because of the blood PH, and ANS changes (pyne, 2004).

Mudras and Bandhas can be described as psychic, emotional, devotional, and aesthetic gestures or attitudes. Yogic have experienced *mudras* as attitudes of energy flow, intended to link individual pranic force with universal or cosmic force (see e.g., figure B 2.3).

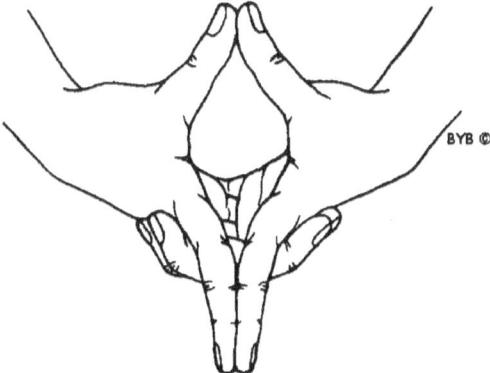

Figure B 2.3. A sample of the Mudras and its psychophysical instructions (quoted from Satyananda 1996, 429-430, with kind permission from Satyananda).

Mudras are a combination of subtle physical movements, which alter mood, attitude, and perception, and with deeper awareness. But *bandhas* aim to loch the pranas in particular areas and redirect their flow into suchumna nadi (the main meridian) for the purpose of spiritual awaking (Satyananda, 1996) (see, e.g., figure B 2.4).

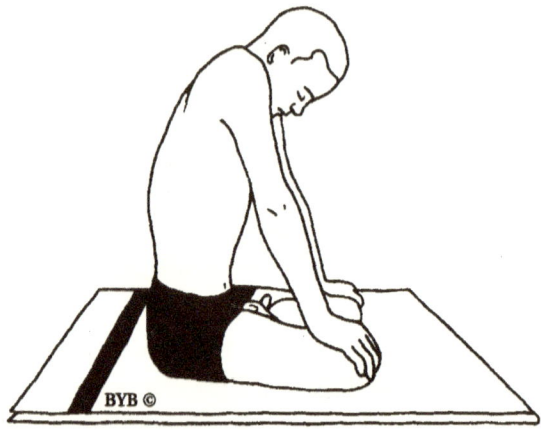

Figure B 2.4. A Sample of the Bandhas and its psychophysical instructions (quoted from Satyananda 1996, 409-411, with kind permission from Satyananda)

Jalandhara Bandha (throat lock)

Sit in padmasana or siddha/siddha yoni asana with the head and spine straight. The knees should be in firm contact with the floor. Those who cannot manage this may perform jalandhara bandha in a standing position.

Place the palms of the hands on the knees.

Close the eyes and relax the whole body.

Inhale slowly and deeply, and retain the breath inside.

While retaining the breath, bend the head forward and press the chin tightly against the chest.

Straighten the arms and lock them firmly into position, pressing the knees down with the hands.

Simultaneously, hunch the shoulders upward and forward.

This will ensure that the arms stay locked, thus intensifying the pressure applied to the neck.

Stay in the final position for as long as the breath can be held comfortably.

Do not strain.

Relax the shoulders, bend the arms, slowly release the lock, raise the head and then exhale.

Repeat when the respiration has returned to normal.

Variation: In kriya yoga a more subtle form of jaland bandha is practiced where the head is simply bent forward so that the chin presses the neck, and the awareness is concentrated on vishuddhi chakra. This kriya variation is the one most commonly used in association with asana practices.

Breathing: The practice may also be performed with external breath retention.

Duration: Jalandhara bandha should be held for as long as the practitioner is able to comfortably retain the breath.

Gradually increase this period by maintaining a count while retaining the breath and increasing the count one by one. This practice may be repeated up to 5 times.

Awareness: Physical—on the throat pit.

Spiritual—on vishuddhi chakra.

Sequence: This bandha is ideally performed in conjunction with pranayamas and mudras. If practiced on its own it should be performed after asanas and pranayamas and before meditation.

Contra-indications: People suffering from cervical spondylosis, high intracranial pressure, vertigo, high blood pressure or heart disease should not practice Jalandhara bandh. Although it reduces blood pressure initially, long retention of the breath brings about some strain on the heart.

Contra-indications: People suffering from cervical spondylosis, high intracranial pressure, vertigo, high blood pressure or heart disease should not practice Jalandhara bandh. Although it reduces blood pressure initially, long retention of the breath brings about some strain on the heart.

Benefits: Jalandhara bandha compresses the carotid sinuses which are located on the carotid arteries, the main arteries in the neck. These sinuses help to regulate the circulatory and respiratory systems. Normally, a decrease of oxygen and increase of carbon dioxide in the body leads to an increased heart rate and heavier breathing. This process is initiated by the carotid sinuses. By artificially exerting pressure on these sinuses, this tendency is prevented, allowing for decreased heart rate and increased breath retention.

This practice produces mental relaxation, relieving stress, anxiety and anger. It develops meditative introversion and one-pointedness. The stimulus on the throat helps to balance thyroid function and regulate the metabolism.

Practice note: Do not inhale or exhale until the chin lock and armlock have been released and the head is fully upright. If any sensation of suffocation is felt, immediately stop and rest. Once the sensation has passed, resume the practice.

Note: *The Sanskrit word* jalan *means 'net' and* dhara *means 'Stream' or 'flow'. One interpretation of jalandhara bandha is the lock which controls the network of nadis in the neck. The physical manifestation of these nadis are the blood vessels and nerves of the neck.*

An alternative definition is that jal *means 'throat',* jalan, *'water' and that* dhara *refers to a tubular vessel in the body. Jalandhara bandha is therefore the throat lock which holds the nectar or fluid flowing down to vishuddhi from bindu and prevents it from falling into the digestive fire. In this way prana is conserved.*

There is also a third meaning. Adhara means 'base' or 'Substratum'. There are sixteen specific centres in the body called adharas which refer to the major and minor chakras. Jalandhara bandha may also be defined as the practice that locks the pranic network of the neck and redirects the flow of subtle energy from this adhara to sushumna nadi in the spine.

Mindfulness Techniques

Yogic mental skills are based on developing of awareness of perceptions, imagination, associations and emotions and leading of these procedures, directly and/or indirectly, in order to release consciousness from the world of multiplicity to the unity. Most of these techniques are experimentally evaluated and standardized as psychotherapeutic techniques in recent decades. Relaxation response, mindfulness meditation, guided imagination and progressive relaxation are some of these reconstructed modern techniques.

Shavasana or physical relaxation is the base of guided imagination and goal-directed visualization techniques of yoga which is named *Yoganidra.*

Witnessing to sensory input such as Auditory or Visual events and concentration training are prepared mind for meditation.

Meditation in its specific definition is pure witnessing to the phenomenological world without any purpose and only for the sake of presence experience and consciousness evolution (Goli, 2008).

In meditation "ego" is externally passive but "self" (as consciousness) is really active and the "organism" is in highest levels of openness.

Meditation almost starts with a mind-body setting (such as meditation asanas, mudras, and imagination) but develops to the no-mind state and egolenness.

Bioenergetic Awareness

Bioenergetic awareness is promoted in advance levels of *asana, pranayama* and the other yogic mind-body interventions, but *kundalini* Yoga is focused specifically on bioenergetic flows (*hadis*), centers (*chakras*) and evoking and controlling of inner bioenergetic resources.

For we never perceive consciousness or thought operative without the vehicle of flesh. It is precisely here that *kundalini* plays a decisive role. As if alive to human aspirations at a certain stage of intellectual development, farsighted nature has planted a divine mechanism in the human body, which by effecting an alteration in the vital energy, or *prana*, feeding the brain, can bring the amazing universe of consciousness within the range of awareness of an awakened man.

The whole science of *kundalini* is based on the manipulation of *Prana-vayu*, the nerve junctions (*cakras*), and the brain. Vayu in Sanskrit means air and the word is used with *prana* to denote its subtle nature. *Prana* and *vayu* are, sometimes, interchangeably used by the ancient authors to designate nerve energy or vital breath. Although *prana* is a self-existent substance, deathless and all-pervading, yet its manifestation in the bodies of terrestrial creatures is rigidly regulated by biological laws. In fact, the whole animal kingdom is the product of the activity of *prana* and the atoms of matter both combined. *Prana* is not something radically different from matter, but both are derivatives from the same basic substance, *Para-shakti* or Primordial Energy (Gopikrishna, 1998).

Each level of the mind is associated with a psychic center, or chakra. The kundalini yoga is to overcome he normal inactivity of the higher chakras so that they are stimulated and the individual is able to experience higher level of the mind. The basic method of awakening these psychic centers in kundalini yoga is deep concentration one the centers and willing their arousal.

A fully awakened kundalini is said actually to restructure the body, leading to a reordering of control over vital functions, such as pulse, intestinal contractions, and brain activity. In hatha yoga, various techniques are used to accomplish this by focusing the life breath or life force (prana) through mental concentration and controlled breathing. Because kundalini is thought to be dormant in the lowest chakra of the energetic body, effort is concentrated on that particular spot (Micozzi & Singh, 2006).

The fourth wave of psychology; transpersonal psychology is deeply inspired of yoga and ancient knowledge of consciousness evolution.

"The whole drift of my education," says Williams James, "goes to I persuade me that the world of our present consciousness is only one out of many worlds of consciousness that exist, and that those other worlds must contain experiences which have a meaning for our life also; and that although in the main their experiences and those of this world keep discrete, yet the two become continuous at certain points, and higher energies filter in. By being faithful in my poor measure to this over-belief, I seem to myself to keep more sane and true. I can, of course, put myself into the sectarian scientist's attitude, and imagine vividly that the world of sensations and of scientific laws and objects may be all. But whenever I do this, I hear that inward monitor . . . whispering the word 'Bosh!' Humbug is humbug, even though it bear the scientific name, and the total expression of human experience, as I view it objectively, invincibly urges me beyond the narrow 'scientific' bounds."

Ken Wilber one of the most effective founders of transpersonal psychology defined the spectrum of consciousness on the base of vibrational anatomy of yoga as shows in figure B 2.5 (Wilber, 1993).

Maya-kosas

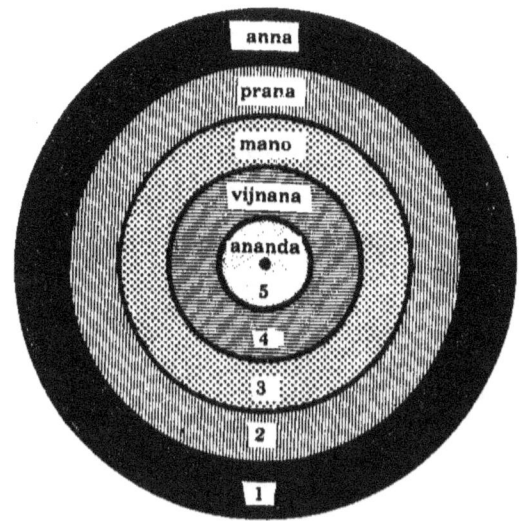

SHEATH	BODY	LEVEL (corresponding)
1. anna-maya-kosa (material)	sthula-sarira (gross)	Ego
2. prana-maya-kosa (vitality)	Suksma-sarira (subtle)	
3. mano-maya-kosa (discrimination)		Existential
4. vijnana-maya-kosa (ratiocination)		
5. ananda-maya-kosa (bliss)	Karana-sarira (causal)	Transpersonal
Brahman—atman		Mind

Figure B 2.5. Yogic vibrational bodies (auras) and levels of consciousness; adapted from Wilber, K. (1993). The spectrum of consciousness.

Anyhow there are various types of Westernized yoga which are simplified and regulated for different purpose such as fitness, stress reduction, wellness, and treatment of physical and mental illness. Several clinical studies show that these mind-body intervention packages can be useful in higher health, but a classic program of yoga can be performed only in the consciousness evolution framework, not as a physical, cognitive-behavioral or bioenergetic technique.

References

Ader, R. & Cohen, N. 1975, "Behaviorally conditioned immunosuppression," *Psychosom Med*, vol. 37, no. 4, pp. 333-340.

Ader, R. & Cohen, N. 1982, "Behaviorally conditioned immunosuppression and murine systemic lupus erythematosus," *Science*, vol. 215, no. 4539, pp. 1534-1536.

Ader, R., Cohen, N., & Felten, D. 1995, "Psychoneuroimmunology: Interactions between the nervous system and the immune system," *Lancet*, vol. 345, no. 8942, pp. 99-103.

Ader, R., Felten, D. L., & Cohen, N. 1991, *Psychoneuroimmunology*, Academic Press, New York.

Adey, W. A. 1990, *Electromagnetic Fields and the Essence of Living Systems. Modern Radio Science*, Oxford University Press, Oxford.

Adey, W. R. & Bawin, S. M. 1977, "Brain interactions with weak electric and magnetic fields," *Neurosci Res Program Bull*, vol. 15, no. 1, pp. 1-129.

Adler, P. A. & Roberts, B. L. 2006, "The use of tai chi to improve health in older adults," *Orthop Nurs*, vol. 25, no. 2, pp. 122-126.

Allais, G., De, L. C., Quirico, P. E., Airola, G., Tolardo, G., Mana, O., & Benedetto, C, 2002, "Acupuncture in the prophylactic treatment of migraine without aura: A comparison with flunarizine," *Headache*, vol. 42, no. 9, pp. 855-861.

Anderson, P. & Anderson, S. A. 1968, *Physiological Basis of the Alpha Rhythm*, Appleton-Century-Crofts, New York.

Arom, K. & MacIntyre, B. "The effect of healing touch on coronary artery bypass surgery patients." Paper presented at Healing Touch International 6th Annual Conference, Denver, 2002.

Ashley, B. & O'Rourke, K. 1994, *Ethics of Health Care: An Introductory Textbook*, Georgetown University Press, Washington DC.

Astin, J., Alternative therapies; Distance healing: Evidence suggests patient may benefit. Obesity, Fitness & Wellness Week 2000.

Astin, J. A, 1997, "Stress reduction through mindfulness meditation. Effects on psychological symptomatology, sense of control, and spiritual experiences," *Psychother Psychosom*, vol. 66, no. 2, pp. 97-106.

Astin, J. A. 1998, "Why patients use alternative medicine: Results of a national study," *JAMA*, vol. 279, no. 19, pp. 1548-1553.

Avants, S. K., Margolin, A., Holford, T. R., & Kosten, T. R. 2000, "A randomized controlled trial of auricular acupuncture for cocaine dependence," *Arch Intern Med*, vol. 160, no. 15, pp. 2305-2312.

Baetz, M. & Toews, J. 2009, "Clinical implications of research on religion, spirituality, and mental health," *Can J Psychiatry*, vol. 54, no. 5, pp. 292-301.

Baggott, A. 1999, *The Encyclopedia of Energy Healing*, Sterling Publisher, New York.

Baginski, B. & Sharamon, Sh. 1988, *Reiki: Universal Life Energy*, Life Rhythm, California.

Baginski, B., Sharamon, Sh., Hanslian, A., Baker, Ch., & Harrison, J. 1997, *Reiki: Universal Life Energy: Holistic Method Suitable for Self-Treatment and the Home Professional Practice, Teleotherapeutics/Spiritual Healing*, New Leaf Distribution Company, New York.

Bajoghli, K., Sharifi, M. & Goli, F. 2003, "Legal Status of Alternative and Complementary Medicine of Iran," *Iranian Journal of Higher Health*, vol. 2, pp. 99-119.

Bar-Yam, Y. 1997, *Dynamics of Complex Systems* Perseus Books, Reading, MA.

Barnes, P., Powell-Griner, E., McFann, K., & Nahm, R. 2002, *CDC Advance Data Report #343: Complementary and Alternative Medicine Use Among Adults*, National Center for Complementary and Alternative Medicine, Washington DC.

Bartlett, J. A., Schleifer, S. J., Demetrikopoulos, M. K., & Keller, S. E. 1995, "Immune differences in children with and without depression," *Biol Psychiatry*, vol. 38, no. 11, pp. 771-774.

Bassett, C. A. 1968, "Biologic significance of piezoelectricity," *Calcif Tissue Res*, vol. 1, no. 4, pp. 252-272.

Bassett, C. A. L. 1978, "Pulsing electromagnetic fields: A new approach to surgical problems," in *Metabolic surgery*, H. Buchwald & R. L. Varco, eds., Grune &Stratton, New York.

Bassett, C. A. L. 1995, "Bioelectromagnetics in the service of medicine," in *Electromagnetic Fields: Biological Interactions and Mechanisms*, M. Blank, ed., American Chemical Society, Washington DC.

Beauchamp, T. L. & Childress, J. F. 1994, *Childress, (1994). Principles of Biomedical Ethics. New York: Oxford University Press*, 4 edn, Oxford University Press, New York.

Beck, R. 1986, "Mood modification with ELF magnetic fields: A preliminary exploration," *Archaeus*, vol. 4, p. 48.

Becker, R. O. 1990, *Cross Currents: The Perils of Electropollution, the Promise of Electromedicine*, Jeremy P Tarcher, Los Angeles.

Becker, R. O. 1991, "Evidence for a primitive DC electrical analog system controlling brain function," *Subtle Energies*, vol. 2, pp. 71-88.

Bell, I. R., Lewis, D. A., Brooks, A. J., Lewis, S. E., & Schwartz, G. E. 2003, "Gas discharge visualization evaluation of ultramolecular doses of homeopathic medicines under blinded, controlled conditions," *J Altern Complement Med*, vol. 9, no. 1, pp. 25-38.

Bell, P., Greene, T., Fisher, J., & Baum, A. 1996, *Environmental Psychology*, Harcourt Brace, Fort Worth.

Bell, R. A., Suerken, C., Quardt, S. A., Grzywacz, J. G., Lang, W., & Arcury, T. A. 2005, "Prayer for health among US adults: The 2002 National Health Interview Survey," *Complementary Health Practice Review*, vol. 10, pp. 175-188.

Benor, D. J. 2000, "Intuitive diagnostics," in *Holistic Nursing: A Handbook for Practice*, 3 edn, B. M. Dossey & L. Keegan, eds., Aspen Publishers, Gaithersburg, MD.

Benson, H. 1976, *The Relaxation Response*, Collins, London.

Benson, H. 1997, *Timeless Healing: The Power and Biology of Belief*, Fireside, New York.

Benveniste, J. From "Water Memory" effects to "Digital Biology" . . . [Cited Jul 2009]. Available from URL: http://www. digibio.com/.

Benveniste, J. From "Water Memory" effects to "Digital Biology" . . . [Cited Jul 2009]. Available from URL: http://www.digibio.com/. 1998.

Berezney, R., Basler, J., Bucholtz, L. A., Smith, H. C., & Siegel, A. J. 1983, Nuclear matrix and DNA replication," in *The Nuclear Envelope and the Nuclear Matrix: Proceedings of the Second Wistar Symposium Held at Sugarloaf Conference Center*, G. G. Maul, ed., A. R. Liss, New York.

Berman, B. M., Singh, B. B., Lao, L., Langenberg, P., Li, H., Hadhazy, V., Bareta, J., & Hochberg, M. 1999, "A randomized trial of acupuncture as an adjunctive therapy in osteoarthritis of the knee," *Rheumatology (Oxford)*, vol. 38, no. 4, pp. 346-354.

Berman, J. D. & Straus, S. E. 2004, "Implementing a research agenda for complementary and alternative medicine," *Annu Rev Med*, vol. 55, pp. 239-254.

Berridge, M. J. & Irvine, R. F. 1989, "Inositol phosphates and cell signalling," *Nature*, vol. 341, no. 6239, pp. 197-205.

Bier, I. D., Wilson, J., Studt, P. & Shakleton, M. 2002, "Auricular acupuncture, education, and smoking cessation: Randomized, sham-controlled trial," *Am J Public Health*, vol. 92, no. 10, pp. 1642-1647.

Birch, S. & Jamison, R. N. 1998, "Controlled trial of Japanese acupuncture for chronic myofascial neck pain: Assessment of specific and nonspecific effects of treatment," *Cli J Pain*, vol. 14, no. 3, pp. 248-255.

Birch, S. I. 1999, *Understanding Acupuncture*, Churchill Livingstone, London.

Birkel, D. A. & Edgren, L. 2000, "Hatha yoga: improved vital capacity of college students," *Altern Ther Health Med*, vol. 6, no. 6, pp. 55-63.

Bohm, D. 1980, *Wholeness and the Implicate Order*, Routledge & Kegan Paul, Boston.

Bouligand, Y. 1978, "Liquid crystals and their analogs in biological systems," *Liquid Crystals*, L. Liebert, ed., Academic Press, New York.

Bovbjerg, D. H., Redd, W. H., Maier, L. A., Holland, J. C., Lesko, L. M., Niedzwiecki, D., Rubin, S. C., & Hakes, T. B. 1990, "Anticipatory immune suppression and nausea in women receiving cyclic chemotherapy for ovarian cancer," *J Consult Clin Psychol*, vol. 58, no. 2, pp. 153-157.

Bradway, C. 1998, "Effects of healing touch on depression," *Healing Touch Newsletter: Research Edition*, vol. 8, no. 3, p. 2.

Brewitt, B. 1996, "Quantities analysis of electrical skin conductance in diagnosis: Historical and current views of bioelectric medicine," *Journal of Naturopathic Medicine*, vol. 6, no. 1, pp. 66-75.

Brewitt, B. 1999, "Electromagnetic medicine and HIV/AIDS treatment: Clinical data and hypothesis for mechanism of action," *AIDS and alternative medicine: The Current State of the Science*, L. J. Standish, C. Calabrese, & M. L. Galation, eds., Harcourt Brace, New York.

Brody, H. 1997, "The physician—patient relationship," in *Medical Ethics*, R. Veatch, ed., Jones & Bartlett Pub, Boston.

Bronzaft, A. L. 2002, "Noise pollution: A hazard to physical and mental well-being," in *Handbook of Environmental Psychology*, R. B. Bechtel & A. Churchman, eds., John Wiley & Sons, New York.

Brovchenko, I., Krukau, A., Oleinikova, A., & Mazur, A. 2007, "Water percolation governs polymorphic transition and conductivity of DNA, from computational biophysics to systems biology (CBSB07)," in *Proceedings of the NIC Workshop 2007*, U. H. E. Hansmann et al., eds., John von Neumann Institute for Computing, Jülich.

Brugh, J. W. 1979, *Joy's Way: A Map for the Transformational Journey*, Tarcher/Putnam, New York.

Burr, H. S. 1972, *Blueprint for Immortality*, The CW Daniel Company, Saffron Walden.

Caldecott, T. Ayurveda: The Divine Science of life. 2006. Philadelphia, Mosby.

Cameron, I. L., Short, N. J., & Fullerton, G. D. 2007, "Verification of simple hydration/ dehydration methods to characterize multiple water compartments on tendon type 1 collagen," *Cell Biol Int*, vol. 31, no. 6, pp. 531-539.

Cameron, M. E. 2001, *Karma and Happiness. A Tibetan Odyssey in Ethics, Spirituality, and Healing*, Fairview Press, Minneapolis, MN.

Campbell, J. 1974, *The Mythic Image*, Princeton University Press, Princeton, NJ.

Cannon, W. B. 1962, *The Wisdom of the Body*, W. W. Norton and Company, Inc., New York.

Capra, F. 2000, *The Tao of Physics: An Exploration of the Parallels between Modern Physics and Eastern Mysticism*, 4 edn, Shambhala Publications, Inc., California.

Carlston, M. 2006 "Homeopathy," in *Fundamentals of Complementary and Alternative Medicine*, M. S. Micozzi, ed., Sunders, Missouri.

Caspi, O. & Bootzin, R. R. 2002, "Evaluating how placebos produce change. Logical and causal traps and understanding cognitive explanatory mechanisms," *Eval Health Prof*, vol. 25, no. 4, pp. 436-464.

Castillo-Richmond, A., Schneider, R. H., Alexander, C. N., Cook, R., Myers, H., Nidich, S., Haney, C., Rainforth, M., & Salerno, J. 2000, "Effects of stress reduction on carotid atherosclerosis in hypertensive African Americans," *Stroke*, vol. 31, no. 3, pp. 568-573.

Chai, Ch. 1975, *The Story of Chinese Philosophy*, Greenwood Press, Westport.

Chang, S. O. 2001, "Meaning of Ki related to touch in caring," *Holist Nurs Pract*, vol. 16, no. 1, pp. 73-84.

Channer, K. S., Barrow, D., Barrow, R., Osborne, M., & Ives, G. 1996, "Changes in haemodynamic parameters following tai chi Chuan and aerobic exercise in patients recovering from acute myocardial infarction," *Postgrad Med J*, vol. 72, no. 848, pp. 349-351.

Chen, K. & Yeung, R. 2002, "Exploratory studies of Qigong therapy for cancer in China," *Integr Cancer Ther*, vol. 1, no. 4, pp. 345-370.

Chen, K. W. & Turner, F. D. 2004, "A case study of simultaneous recovery from multiple physical symptoms with medical Qigong therapy," *J Altern Complement Med*, vol. 10, no. 1, pp. 159-162.

Chien, C. H., Tsuei, J. J., Lee, S. C., Huang, Y. C., & Wei, Y. H. 1991b, "Effect of emitted bioenergy on biochemical functions of cells," *Am J Chin Med*, vol. 19, no. 3-4, pp. 285-292.

Chien, C. H., Tsuei, J. J., Lee, S. C., Huang, Y. C., & Wei, Y. H. 1991a, "Effect of emitted bioenergy on biochemical functions of cells," *Am J Chin Med*, vol. 19, no. 3-4, pp. 285-292.

Chopra, D. 1990, *Quantum Healing: Exploring the Frontiers of Mind/Body Medicine*, Bantam, New York.

Chopra, D. 1994, "Keynote lecture at Columbia University Dharam Minduja Indic Research Center Conference," *J Altern Complement Med*, vol. 1, no. 3, pp. 247-301.

Choy, R. Y. S., Monro, J. A., & Smith, C. W. 1987, "Electrical sensitivities in allergy patients," *Clinical Ecology*, vol. 4, no. 3, pp. 93-102.

Collinge, W., Wentworth, R. & Sabo, S. 2005, "Integrating complementary therapies into community mental health practice: An exploration," *J Altern Complement Med*, vol. 11, no. 3, pp. 569-574.

Connor, K. M., Davidson, J. R., & Lee, L. C. 2003, "Spirituality, resilience, and anger in survivors of violent trauma: a community survey," *J Trauma Stress*, vol. 16, no. 5, pp. 487-494.

Conveney, P. & Highfield, R. 1995, *Frontiers of Complexity: The Search for Order in a Chaotic World*, Ballantine Publishing Group, New York.

Corn-Becker, F., Welch, l. & Fisichelli, V. 1949, "Conditioning factors underlying hypnosis," *J Abnorm Psychol*, vol. 44, no. 2, pp. 212-222.

Corongiu, G. & Clementi, E. 1981, "Simulations of the solvent structure for macromolecules. II. Structure of water solvating Na+-B-DNa at 300 K and a model for conformational transitions induced by solvent variations," *Biopolymers*, vol. 20, pp. 2427-2483.

Coughlin, P. 2002, "Manual Therapies," in *Fundamentals of Complementary and Alternative Medicine*, M. S. Micozzal, ed., Churchill Livingston, Edinburgh.

Crasilneck, H. B. & Hall, J. A. 1985, *Clinical Hypnosis: Principles and Applications*, Grune & Stratton, New York.

Crawford, C. C., Spparber, A. G., & Janis, W. B. 2003, "A systematic review of the quality of research on hand-on and distance healing: Clinical and laboratory studies," *Alternative Therapies in Health and Medicine*, vol. 9, no. 3, pp. 96-106.

Crawford, SE., Leaver, V. W., & Mahoney, S. D. 2006, "Using Reiki to decrease memory and behavior problems in mild cognitive impairment and mild Alzheimer's disease," *J Altern Complement Med*, vol. 12, no. 9, pp. 911-913.

Cutler, R. G. 2005, "Oxidative stress profiling: part I. Its potential importance in the optimization of human health," *Ann N Y Acad Sci*, vol. 1055, pp. 93-135.

D'Aprile, J. 2002, "Energy Medicine," in *Complementary and Alternative Medicine Secrets*, W. Kohatsu, ed., Hanley & Belfus, Philadelphia.

Dacher, E. 2006, "Integrated medical model," in *Fundamental of Complementary and Alternative Medicine*, M. S. Micozzi, ed., Saunders, Philadelphia.

Dadsetan, B. 1997, *Developmental Pathopsychology*, Samt, Tehran.

Davis, W. B., Thaut, H. M., & Gfeller, K. E. 1998, *An Introduction to Music Therapy: Theory and Practice* McGraw, Hill Humanities, New York.

Deleuze, G. & Guattari, F. 1987, *A Thousand Plateaus: Capitalism and Schizophrenia*, University of Minnesota Press, Minneapolis, MN.

Denison, B. 2004, "Touch the pain away: New research on therapeutic touch and persons with fibromyalgia syndrome," *Holist Nurs Pract*, vol. 18, no. 3, pp. 142-151.

Destexhe, A., Babloyantz, A., & Sejnowski, T. J. 1993, "Ionic mechanisms for intrinsic slow oscillations in thalamic relay neurons," *Biophys J*, vol. 65, no. 4, pp. 1538-1552.

Dhonden, Y. 2000, *Healing from the Source: The Science and Lore of Tibetan Medicine*, Snow Lion Publications, Ithaca, NY.

Diener, D. 2001, "A pilot study of the effect of chakra connection and magnetic unruffle on perception of pain in people with fibromyalgia," *Healing Touch Newsletter: Research Edition*, vol. 10, no. 3, pp. 7-8.

Dilts, R., Hallbom, T., & Smith, S. 1991, *Beliefs: Pathways to Health and Wellbeing*, Metamorphous Press, New York.

Discepolo, C. 2009, *Lunar Returns and Earth Returns: Two Supporting Methodologies of Active Astrology*, Ricerca, Naples.

Donough-Means, S. I., Kreitzer, M. J., & Bell, I. R. 2004, "Fostering a healing presence and investigating its mediators," *J Altern Complement Med*, vol. 10 Suppl 1, p. S25-S41.

Dossey, B., Keegan, L., Guzzetta, C., & Kolkmeier, L. 1995, *Holistic Nursing: A Handbook for Practice*, Jones & Bartlett Publishers, Sudbury, MA.

Dossey, L. 1996, *Human Nature and Conduct*, Henry Holt and Company, New York.

Dresser, L. J. & Singh, S. 1997, "Effects of Reiki on pain and selected affective and personality variables of chronically ill patients," *Subtle Energies*, vol. 9, pp. 51-82.

Duerden, T. 2004, "An aura of confusion Part 2: The aided eye—'imaging the aura?'," *Complement Ther Nurs Midwifery*, vol. 10, no. 2, pp. 116-123.

Dunlap, J. C., Loros, J. J., & Decoursey, P. J. 2003, *Chronobiology, biological time keeping*, Sinauer Associates Inc., Massachusetts.

Dunne, B. J. & Jahn, R. G. 1987, *Margins of Reality: The Role of Consciousness in the Physical World*, Harcourt Brace, New York.

Dziemidko, H. E. 1999, *The Complete Book of Energy Medicine*, Gaia Books Limited, London.

Eckes Peck, S. D. 1997, "The effectiveness of therapeutic touch for decreasing pain in elders with degenerative arthritis," *J Holist Nurs*, vol. 15, no. 2, pp. 176-198.

Edwards, D. L. 1991, "A meta-analysis of the effects of meditation and hypnosis on measures of anxiety," *Dissert Abstr Int*, vol. 52, no. 2-B, pp. 1039-1040.

Eliade, M. 1964, *Shamanism: Archaic Techniques of Ecstasy*, Princeton University Press, Princeton.

Ellison, J. & Garrod, D. R. 1984, "Anchoring filaments of the amphibian epidermal-dermal junction traverse the basal lamina entirely from the plasma membrane of hemidesmosomes to the dermis," *J Cell Sci*, vol. 72, pp. 163-172.

Enander, B. & Larson, G. 1977, "Microwave radiometric measurements of the temperature inside a body," *Electronic Letter*, vol. 10, p. 317.

Endler, P. C. & Schulte, J. 1994, *Ultra High Dilution: Physiology and Physics*, Springer, Dordrecht.

Engel, G. L. 1980, "The clinical application of the biopsychosocial model," *Am. J Psychiatry*, vol. 137, no. 5, pp. 535-544.

Ernst, E. 2003, "Distant healing—an 'update' of a systematic review," *Wien Klin Wochenschr*, vol. 115, no. 7-8, pp. 241-245

Ernst, E. & Resch, K. L. 1995, "Concept of true and perceived placebo effects," *BMJ*, vol. 311, no. 7004, pp. 551-553.

Esgate, A. E. & Groome, D. 2001, "Probability and coincidence," in *Parapsychology: The Science of Unusual Experience*, R. Roberts & D. Groome, eds., Oxford University Press, Oxford.

Evans, D. L., Folds, J. D., Petitto, J. M., Golden, R. N., Pedersen, C. A., Corrigan, M., Gilmore, J. H., Silva, S. G., Quade, D., & Ozer, H. 1992, "Circulating natural killer cell phenotypes in men and women with major depression. Relation to cytotoxic activity and severity of depression," *Arch Gen Psychiatry*, vol. 49, no. 5, pp. 388-395.

Fellows, L. E. 1997, "Opening up the 'black box,'" *International Journal of Alternative and Complementary Medicine*, vol. 15, no. 8, pp. 9-13.

Ferrucci, P. 1983, *What We May Be*, Turnstone Press, Wellingborough.

Fiol, C. M. & O'Connor, E. J. 2004, "The power of mind: What if the game is bigger than we think," *Journal of Management Inquiry*, vol. 13, no. 4, pp. 342-352.

Fis, A. M. Reiki, La Voie Des 5 Prinsipes. 1998. Suisse, Recto verseau.

Foster, K. R. & Pickard, W. F. 1987, "Microwaves: The risks of risk research," *Nature*, vol. 330, pp. 531-532.

Foucault, M. 1994, *The Birth of the Clinic: An Archaeology of Medical Perception*, Vintage Books, New York.

Frawley, D. 1997, *Ayurvedic Healing: A Comprehensive Guides*, Motilal Banarsidass Publishers, Delhi.

Friedman, H., Becker, R. O., & Bachman, C. 1965, "Psychiatric ward behavior and geophysical parameters," *Nature*, vol. 205, pp. 1050-1052.

Frohlich, H. F. 1988, *Biological Coherence and Response to External Stimuli*, Springer, Berlin.

Gallagher, R. & Appenzeller, T. 1999, "Beyond reductionism," *Science*, vol. 284, p. 79.

Gallo, F. 1998, *Energy Psychology*, CRC Press, Boca Raton, FL.

Gallo, F. 1999, *Innovations in Psychology*, CRC Press, Boca Raton, FL.

Gallo, F. P. 2002, *Energy Psychology in Psychotherapy: A Comprehensive Source Book*, W. W. Norton, New York.

Gardner, D. 1985, "Presence," in *Nursing Interventions: Treatments for Nursing Diagnoses*, G. Bulechek & J. McCloskey, eds., Saunders, Philadelphia.

Garfinkel, M. & Schumacher, H. R. Jr. 2000, "Yoga," *Rheum Dis Clin North Am*, vol. 26, no. 1, pp. 125-32, x.

Garfinkel, M. S., Schumacher, H. R. Jr., Husain, A., Levy, M., & Reshetar, R. A. 1994, "Evaluation of a yoga based regimen for treatment of osteoarthritis of the hands," *J Rheumatol*, vol. 21, no. 12, pp. 2341-2343.

Garfinkel, M. S., Singhal, A., Katz, W. A., Allan, D. A., Reshetar, R., & Schumacher, H. R. Jr. 1998, "Yoga-based intervention for carpal tunnel syndrome: A randomized trial," *JAMA*, vol. 280, no. 18, pp. 1601-1603.

Garrard, C. T. 1995, "The effect of therapeutic touch on stress reduction and immune function in persons with AIDS," *Dissertation Abstracts Int*, vol. 56, no. 3692B, p., University Microfilms #9537117.

Geggus, P. 2004, "Introduction to the concepts of zero balancing, journal of bodywork and movement therapies, 8:58-71," *Journal of Bodywork and Movement Therapies*, vol. 8, no. 1, pp. 58-71.

Gehlhaart, C. & Dail, P. 2000, "Effectiveness of healing touch and therapeutic touch on elderly residents of long-term care facilities on reducing pain and anxiety levels," *Healing Touch Newsletter*, vol. 0, no. 3, p. 8.

Gerber, R. 1988, *Vibrational Medicine*, Bear & Company, Santa Fe, NM.

Gifford, R. 2007, *Environmental Psychology: Principles and Practice*, Optimal Books, Colville.

Glaser, R., Kiecolt-Glaser, J. K., Malarkey, W. B., & Sheridan, J. "The effect of stress on viral vaccine responses," in *International Symposium of Psychoneuroimmunoendocrinology*, Buenos Aires.

Golembiewski, R., Billingsley, K., & Yeager, S. 1976, "Measuring change and persistence in human affairs: Types of change generated by OD designs," *Journal of Applied Behavioral Science*, vol. 12, pp. 133-157.

Goli, F. 2003a, "An Introduction to Integrative Medicine: New domains for ancient wisdom examination," *Iranian Journal of Higher Health (Salamat-e-Bartar)*, vol. 1, no. 1, pp. 3-45.

Goli, F. 2003b, "Yoga: An ancient paradigm of biopsychosocial model," *Iranian Journal of Higher Health*.

Goli, F. 2004, "An essay on psychoanalysis of illness experience," *Iranian Journal of Higher Health (Salamat-e-Bartar)*, vol. 4, no. 5, pp. 95-107.

Goli, F. 2008, "Clinical analysis of energy-information flow in therapist-client communication," *Iranian Journal of Higher Health*, vol. 7, pp. 7-21.

Goodman, A. 1991, "Organic unity theory: The mind-body problem revisited," *Am J Psychiatry*, vol. 148, no. 5, pp. 553-563.

Gordon, D. 1978, *Therapeutic Metaphors: Helping Others Through the Looking Glass*, Meta Publications, California.

Greenfield, R. H. 2002, "Yoga," in *Complementary and Alternative Medicine Secrets*, W. Kohatsu, ed., Hanley & Belfus, Philadelphia.

Grinderg-Zylberberbanm, J., Delaflor, M., Attie, L., & Goswami, A. 1994, "The Einstein-Podolsky-Rosen paradox in the brain the transferred potential," *Physics Essays*, vol. 7, no. 4, pp. 422-428.

Grinderg-Zylberberbanm, J., Delaflor, M., Sanchez, M. E., Guevara, M. A., & Perez, M. 1992, "Human communication and the electrophysiological activity of the brain.," *Subtle Energies*, vol. 3, no. 3, pp. 25-43.

Grof, S. 1972, "Varieties of transpersonal experiences: Observations from LSD psychotherapy," *Journal of Transpersonal Psychology*, vol. 4, no. 1, pp. 45-80.

Groome, D. 2001, "Astrology," in *Parapsychology: The Science of unusual experience*, R. Roberts & D. Groome, eds., Arnold, New York.

Gross, R., Sasson, Y., Zarhy, M. & Zohar, J. 1998, "Healing environment in psychiatric hospital design," *Gen Hosp Psychiatry*, vol. 20, no. 2, pp.108-114.

Gueldner, S. H., Michel, Y., Bramlett, M. H., Liu, C. F., Johnston, L. W., Endo, E., Minegishi, H., & Carlyle, M. S. 2005, "The well-being picture scale: a revision of the index of field energy," *Nurs Sci Q*, vol. 18, no. 1, pp. 42. 42-50.

Guevara, E., Menidas, N., & Suva, C. 2002, *Developing a Protocol for Decreasing Post Traumatic Stress Symptoms in Abused Women. Paper Presented at the 8th Nursing Research Pan American Colloquium, Mexico City*.

Guy, A. W., Chou, C. K., Lin, J. C., & Christensen, D. 1975, "Microwave-induced acoustic effects in mammalian auditory systems and physical materials," *Ann N Y Acad Sci*, vol. 247, pp. 194-218.

Habermas, I. 1984, *The Theory of Communicative Action. Reason and Tire Rationalization of Society*, Heinemann, London.

Hall, H., Minnes, L., & Olness, K. 1993, "The psychophysiology of voluntary immunomodulation," *Int J Neurosci*, vol. 69, no. 1-4, pp. 221-234.

Hall, H., Papas, A., Tosi, M., & Olness, K. 1996, "Directional changes in neutrophil adherence following passive resting versus active imagery," *Int J Neurosci*, vol. 85, no. 3-4, pp. 185-194.

Hall, J. A., Woodman, M., Stein, M., Goodheart, W. B., Machtiger, H. G., Beebe, J., Meador, B. D. Sh., Wiedeman, F. L., & Salant, N. S. 1984, *Chiron: Transference/Countertransference*, Chiron Publications, New York.

Hall, M. Reiki for the Soul. 2000. London, Thorsons.

Halperin, E. C. 2001, "Should academic medical centers conduct clinical trials of the efficacy of intercessory prayer?" *Acad Med*, vol. 76, no. 8, pp. 791-797.

Hammond, D. C. 1990, *Handbook of Hypnotic Suggestions and Metaphors*, WW Norton & Co., New York.

Hanser, S. B. 2000, *The New Music Therapist's Handbook*, 2 edn, Berklee Press Publications, Boston.

Harrington, A. 1997, *The Placebo Effect: An Interdisciplinary Exploration*, Harvard University Press, Cambridge.

Hartig, T., Evans, G. W., Jamner, L. D., Davis, D. S., & Garling, T. 2003, "Tracking restoration in natural and urban field settings," *J Environ Psychol*, vol. 23, pp. 109-123.

Haslam, R. 2001, "A comparison of acupuncture with advice and exercises on the symptomatic treatment of osteoarthritis of the hip—A randomised controlled trial," *Acupunct Med*, vol. 19, no. 1, pp. 19-26.

Hay, E. D. 1981a, *Cell Biology of Extracellular Matrix*, Plenum, New York.

Hay, E. D. 1981b, "Extracellular matrix," *Journal of Cell Biology*, vol. 91, pp. 205s—223s.

Hay, L. L. 1988, *You Can Heal Your Life*, Specialist Printing, Concord, MA.

Heidt, P. 1981, "Effect of therapeutic touch on anxiety level of hospitalized patients," *Nurs Res*, vol. 30, no. 1, pp. 32-37.

Herbert, N. 1994, *Elemental Mind: Human Consciousness and the New Physics*, Plume, New York.

Heron-Marx, S., Price-Knol, F., Burden, B., & Hicks, C. 2008, "A systematic Review of the Use of Reiki in Health Care," *Alternative and Complementary Therapies*, vol. 2, pp. 37-42.

Hintz, K. J., Yount, G. L., Kadar, I., Schwartz, G., Hammerschlag, R., & Lin, S. 2003, "Bioenergy definitions and research guidelines," *Altern Ther Health Med*, vol. 9, no. 3 Suppl, p. A13-A30.

Ho, M. W. & Knight, D. P. 1998, "The acupuncture system and the liquid crystalline collagen fibers of the connective tissues," *Am J Chin Med*, vol. 26, no. 3-4, pp. 251-263.

Ho, M. W., Popp, F. A. & Warnke, U. 1994, *Bioelectrodynamics and biocommunication*, World Scientific, Singapore.

Hodge, D. R. 2007, "A Systematic Review of the Empirical Literature on Intercessory Prayer," *Research on Social Work Practice*, vol. 17, no. 2, pp. 174-187.

Horwitz, A. F. 1997, "Integrins and Health," *Scientific American*, vol. 276, pp. 68-75.

Hover-Kramer, D. 1989, "Creating a context for self-healing: The transpersonal perspective," *Holist Nurs Pract*, vol. 3, no. 3, pp. 27-34.

Hover-Kramer, D. 1996, *Healing Touch: A Resource for Health-Care Professionals*, Delmar Publishers, New York.

Hurwitz, W. 2001, "Energy medicine," in *Fundamentals of Complementary and Alternative Medicine*, 2 edn, M. S. Micozzi, ed., Churchill Livingstone, New York.

Ibison, M. & Haisch, B. 1996, "Quantum and classical statistics of the electromagnetic zero-point field," *Phys Rev A*, vol. 54, no. 4, pp. 2737-2744.

Ina, V. S. & Chrisman, L. 2001, "Massage and Bodywork," in *Integrating Complementary Medicine into Health Systems*, M. Faass, ed., Aspen Publication, Marylan.

Ingber, D. E. 1993, "Cellular tensegrity: Defining new rules of biological design that govern the cytoskeleton," *J Cell Sci*, vol. 104 (Pt 3), pp. 613-627.

Ingber, D. E. 1998, "The architecture of life," *Sci Am*, vol. 278, no. 1, pp. 48-57.

Ingerman, S. 1991, *Soul Retrieval: Mending the Fragmented Self Through Shamanic Practice*, Harper Collins, San Francisco.

Irigaray, L. 2000, *To Be Two*, The Athlone Press, London.

Irwin, M., Patterson, T., Smith, T. L., Caldwell, C., Brown, S. A., Gillin, J. C., & Grant, I. 1990, "Reduction of immune function in life stress and depression," *Biol Psychiatry*, vol. 27, no. 1, pp. 22-30.

Jackson, J. D. 1975, *Classical Electrodynamics*, Wiley, New York.

Jackson, M. & Mantasch, H. H. 1996, "Biomedical infrared spectroscopy," in *Infrared Spectroscopy of Biomolecules*, H. H. Mantsch & D. Chapman, eds., Wiley, New York.

Jacobs, J. & Moskowitz, R. 2002, "Homeopathy," in *Fundamentals of complementary and alternative medicine*, M. S. Micozzi, ed., Churchill Livingston, Edinburgh.

Jacobs, J. A. 1987, *Geomagnetism*, Academic Press, London.

Jacobson, E. 1978, *You Must Relax: Practical Methods for Reducing the Tensions of Modern Living*, Souvenir Press, London.

Jahn, R. G. 2001, "The Challenge of Consciousness," *Journal of Scientific Explorations*, vol. 15, no. 4, pp. 443-457.

Jahn, R. G. & Dunne, B. J. 1986, "On the Quantum Mechanics of Consciousness, With Application to Anomalous Phenomena," *Foundations of Physics*, vol. 16, no. 8, pp. 721-772.

Janakiramaiah, N., Gangadhar, B. N., Naga Venkatesha Murthy, P. J., Harish, M. G., Subbakrishna, D. K., & Vedamurthachar, A. 2000, "Antidepressant efficacy of Sudarshan Kriya Yoga (SKY) in melancholia: a randomized comparison with electroconvulsive therapy (ECT) and imipramine," *J Affect Disord*, vol. 57, no. 1-3, pp. 255-259.

Jang, H. S., Lee, M. S., Kim, M. J., & Chong, E. S. 2004, "Effects of Qi therapy on premenstrual syndrome," *Int J Neurosci*, vol. 114, no. 8, pp. 909-921.

Jasnoski, M. B. 1992, "The physical environment affects quality of life based upon environmental sensitivity," *Journal of Applied Developmental Psychology*, vol. 13, pp. 139-142.

Johari, H. 1987, *Chakras: Energy Centers of Transformation*, Destiny Books, Rochester.

Johnston, J. & Barcan, R. 2006, "Subtle transformations: Imaging the body in alternative health practices," *International Journal of Cultural Studies*, vol. 9, no. 1, pp. 25-44.

Jonas, W. B. & Crawford, C. C. 2003, "Science and spiritual healing: A critical review of spiritual healing, 'energy' medicine, and intentionality," *Altern Ther Health Med*, vol. 9, no. 2, pp. 56-61.

Joos, S., Schott, C., Zou, H., Daniel, V. & Martin, E. 2000, "Immunomodulatory effects of acupuncture in the treatment of allergic asthma: a randomized controlled study," *J Altern Complement Med*, vol. 6, no. 6, pp. 519-525.

Kabat-Zinn, J., Wheeler, E., Light, T., Skillings, A., Scharf, M. J., Cropley, T. G., Hosmer, D., & Bernhard, J. D. 1998, "Influence of a mindfulness meditation-based stress reduction intervention on rates of skin clearing in patients with moderate to severe psoriasis undergoing phototherapy (UVB) and photochemotherapy (PUVA)," *Psychosom Med*, vol. 60, no. 5, pp. 625-632.

Kay, R. W. 1994, "Geomagnetic storms: association with incidence of depression as measured by hospital admission," *Br J Psychiatry*, vol. 164, no. 3, pp. 403-409.

Keller, E. & Bzdek, V. M. 1986, "Effects of therapeutic touch on tension headache pain," *Nurs Res*, vol. 35, no. 2, pp. 101-106.

Kemp, C. 2004, "Qigong as a therapeutic intervention with older adults," *Journal of Holistic Nursing*, vol. 4, pp. 351-373.

Kiang, J. G., Ives, J. A., & Jonas, W. B. 2005, "External bioenergy-induced increases in intracellular free calcium concentrations are mediated by Na+/Ca2+ exchanger and L-type calcium channel," *Mol Cell Biochem*, vol. 271, no. 1-2, pp. 51-59.

Kiang, J. G., Koenig, M. L., & Smallridge, R. C. 1992, "Heat shock increases cytosolic free Ca2+ concentration via Na(+)-Ca2+ exchange in human epidermoid A 431 cells," *Am J Physiol*, vol. 263, no. 1 Pt 1, p. C30-C38.

Kiang, J. G., Marotta, D., Wirkus, M., Wirkus, M., & Jonas, W. B. 2002, "External bioenergy increases intracellular free calcium concentration and reduces cellular response to heat stress," *J Investig Med*, vol. 50, no. 1, pp. 38-45.

Kiang, J. G. & Smallridge, R. C. 1994, "Sodium cyanide increases cytosolic free calcium: Evidence for activation of the reversed mode of the Na+/Ca2+ exchanger and Ca2+ mobilization from inositol trisphosphate-insensitive pools," *Toxicol Appl Pharmacol*, vol. 127, no. 2, pp. 173-181.

Kiang, J. G. & Tsokos, G. C. 1998, "Heat shock protein 70 kDa: Molecular biology, biochemistry, and physiology," *Pharmacol Ther*, vol. 80, no. 2, pp. 183-201.

Kiecolt-Glaser, J. K., Glaser, R., Strain, E. C., Stout, J. C., Tarr, K. L., Holliday, J. E., & Speicher, C. E. 1986, "Modulation of cellular immunity in medical students," *J Behav Med*, vol. 9, no. 1, pp. 5-21.

Kim, S. J. Condition, pattern, and consequences of Ki support of the Korean elderly. University of California San Francisco, Doctoral Dissertation. 1995.

Kim, T. 2004, "The concept of magnetism from a Rogerian perspective," *Theoria, Journal of Nursing Theory*, vol. 13, pp. 4-9.

Kirsch, I. & Sapirstein, G. 1998, "Listening to Prozac but Hearing Placebo: A Meta-Analysis of Antidepressant Medication," *Prevention & Treatment*, vol. 1, no. 2, p. article 0002a.

Kirsteins, A. E., Dietz, F., & Hwang, S. M. 1991, "Evaluating the safety and potential use of a weight-bearing exercise, Tai-Chi Chuan, for rheumatoid arthritis patients," *Am J Phys Med Rehabil*, vol. 70, no. 3, pp. 136-141.

Kleijnen, J., Knipschild, P. & ter, R. G. 1991, "Clinical trials of homoeopathy," *BMJ*, vol. 302, no. 6772, pp. 316-323.

Knight, B., Mudge, C., Openshaw, S., White, A., & Hart, A. 2001, "Effect of acupuncture on nausea of pregnancy: A randomized, controlled trial," *Obstet Gynecol*, vol. 97, no. 2, pp. 184-188.

Koenig, H. G., McCullough, M. E., & Larson, D. B. 2001, *Handbook of Religion and Health*, Oxford University Press, New York.

Kohatsu, W. 2002, *Complementary and Alternative Medicine Secrets*, Hanley & Belfus, Philadelphia.

Koithan, M., Bell, I. R., Caspi, O., Ferro, L., & Brown, V. 2007, "Patients' experiences and perceptions of a consultative model integrative medicine clinic: a qualitative study," *Integr Cancer Ther*, vol. 6, no. 2, pp. 174-184.

Korpela, K. M., Klemettila, T., & Hietanen, J. K. 2002, "Evidence for rapid affective evaluation of environmental scenes," *Environment and Behavior*, vol. 34, pp. 634-650.

Kosko, B. 2001, *Fuzzy Thinking: The New Science of Fuzzy Logic*, Hyperion, New York.

Krieger, D. 1979, *Therapeutic Touch: How to Use Your Hands to Help or to Heal*, Simon & Schuster, New York.

Krippner, S. 1995, "A Cross-Cultural Comparison of Four Healing Models," *Altern Ther Health Med*, vol. 1, no. 1, pp. 22-29.

Krischenbaum, H. & Henderson, V. 1990, *The Carl Rogers Reader*, Constable, London.

Krishna, G. 1972, *The Biological Basis of Religion and Genius*, Harpercollins Publisher, New York.

Krishna, G. 1978, *The Biological Basis of Religion and Genius*, Harpercollins Publisher, New York.

Krishna, G. 2000, *Kundalini: The Secret of Yoga*, Institute for Consciousness Research, Ontario.

Krucoff, M. W., Crater, S. W., Green, C. L., Maas, A. C., Seskevich, J. E., Lane, J. D., Loeffler, K. A., Morris, K., Bashore, T. M., & Koenig, H. G. 2001, "Integrative noetic therapies as adjuncts to percutaneous intervention during unstable coronary syndromes: Monitoring and Actualization of Noetic Training (MANTRA) feasibility pilot," *Am Heart J*, vol. 142, no. 5, pp. 760-769.

Kuang, A., Wang, C., Xu, D., & Qian, Y. 1991, "Research on 'anti-aging' effect of Qigong," *J Tradit Chin Med*, vol. 11, no. 2, pp. 153-158.

Kumar, R. A. & Kurup, P. A. 2003, "Changes in the isoprenoid pathway with transcendental meditation and Reiki healing practices in seizure disorder," *Neurol India*, vol. 51, no. 2, pp. 211-214.

Kunz, D. & Peper, E. 1982, "Fields and their clinical implications," *American Theosophist*, vol. 70, pp. 395-401.

Lauffenburger, D. A. & Horwitz, A. F. 1996, "Cell migration: A physically integrated molecular process," *Cell*, vol. 84, no. 3, pp. 359-369.

Laumann, K., Carling, T., & Stormark, K. M. 2003, "Selective attention and heart rate responses to natural and urban environments," *Journal of Environmental Psychology*, vol. 23, pp. 125-134.

Leddy, S. K. 1998, *Leddy and Pepper's Conceptual bases of Professional Nursing*, Lippincott Williams & Wilkins, Philadelphia.

Leddy, S. K. 2004, "Human energy: A conceptual model of unitary nursing science," *Visions: The Journal of Rogerian Science*, vol. 12, no. 1, pp. 14-27.

Leddy, S. K. 2006, *Integrative Health Promotion: Conceptual Bases for Nursing Practice*, Jones and Bartlett Publishers, Boston.

Lee, M. S., Jang, J. W., Jang, H. S., & Moon, S. R. 2003, "Effects of Qi therapy on blood pressure, pain and psychological symptoms in the elderly: a randomized controlled pilot trial," *Complement Ther Med*, vol. 11, no. 3, pp. 159-164.

Lee, M. S., Pittler, M. H., & Ernst, E. 2008, "Effects of Reiki in clinical practice: A systematic review of randomised clinical trials," *Int J Clin Pract*, vol. 62, no. 6, pp. 947-954.

Leonidov, I. 1962, *Signals of What? Soviet Union 145*, Kirov State University, Alma-Ata.

Levin, J. 2003, "Spiritual determinants of health and healing: an epidemiologic perspective on salutogenic mechanisms," *Altern Ther Health Med*, vol. 9, no. 6, pp. 48-57.

Levin, J. 2008, "Esoteric healing traditions: A conceptual overview," *Explore (NY)*, vol. 4, no. 2, pp. 101-112.

Levin, J. & Mead, L. 2008, "Bioenergy healing: A theoretical model and case series," *Explore (NY)*, vol. 4, no. 3, pp. 201-209.

Liboff, A. R., Williams, T. Jr., Strong, D. M., & Wistar, R. Jr. 1984, "Time-varying magnetic fields: Effect on DNA synthesis," *Science*, vol. 223, no. 4638, pp. 818-820.

Liguori, A., Petti, F., Bangrazi, A., Camaioni, D., Guccione, G., Pitari, G. M., Bianchi, A., & Nicoletti, W. E. 2000, "Comparison of pharmacological treatment versus acupuncture treatment for migraine without aura—analysis of socio-medical parameters," *J Tradit Chin Med*, vol. 20, no. 3, pp. 231-240.

Ling, G. N. 1992, *A Revolution in the Physiology of the Living Cell*, Krieger Publishing Company, Malabar.

Little, S. 2004, "Mind-Body Medicine," in *Integrative Medicine; Principles for Practice*, B. Kligler & R. Lee, eds., McGraw-Hill, New York.

Locke, S. E., Ransil, B. J., Zachariae, R., Molay, F., Tollins, K., Covino, N. A., & Danforth, D. 1994, "Effect of hypnotic suggestion on the delayed-type hypersensitivity response," *JAMA*, vol. 272, no. 1, pp. 47-52.

Loh, S. H. 1999, "Qigong therapy in the treatment of metastatic colon cancer," *Altern Ther Health Med*, vol. 5, no. 4, pp. 112, 111.

Luebeck, W. 1991, *Aura Healing Handbook*, Lotus Press, Shangri.

MacDermott, W. E. & Epstein, M. Reiki is effective in addressing major consequences of child sexual abuse, 2001. [cited Jan 12, 2006]. Available from URL: www.tamarashouse.sk.ca/reiki.pdf.

MacDermott, W. E. & Epstein, M. Reiki is effective in addressing major consequences of child sexual abuse, 2001. [cited Jan 12, 2006]. Available from URL: www.tamarashouse. sk.ca/reiki.pdf.

MacDermott, W. E. & Epstein, M. Reiki is effective in addressing major consequences of child sexual abuse, 2001. [cited Jan 12, 2006]. Available from URL: www.tamarashouse. sk.ca/reiki.pdf. 2006.

MacGinitie, L. A. 1995, "Streaming and piezoelectric potentials in connective tissues," in *Electromagnetic Fields: Biological Interactions and Mechanisms*, M. Blank, ed., American Chemical Society, Washington DC.

Mackay, N., Hansen, S. & McFarlane, O. 2004, "Autonomic nervous system changes during Reiki treatment: a preliminary study," *J Altern Complement Med*, vol. 10, no. 6, pp. 1077-1081.

Mackean, D. G. 1973, *Introduction to biology* John Murray Ltd., London.

MacNeil, M. S. 2006, "Therapeutic touch, pain, and caring: Implications for nursing practice," *International Journal for Human Caring*, vol. 10, pp. 40-48.

Mansour, A. A., Beuche, M., Laing, G., Leis, A., & Nurse, J. 1999, "A study to test the effectiveness of placebo Reiki standardization procedures developed for a planned Reiki efficacy study," *J Altern Complement Med*, vol. 5, no. 2, pp. 153-164.

Maslow, A. H. 1970, *Religions, Values, and Peak-Experiences*, The Viking Press, New York.

Masters, K. S. & Spielmans, G. I. 2007, "Prayer and health: Review, meta-analysis, and research agenda," *J Behav Med*, vol. 30, no. 4, pp. 329-338.

Mathews, A. P. 1903, "Electrical polarity in the hydroids," *Am J Physiol*, vol. 8, pp. 294-299.

Matsumoto, K. & Birch, S. 1988, *Hara Diagnosis: Reflections on the Sea*, Paradigm Pubs, Brookline.

McKenzie, E. 1998, *Healing Reiki*, Ulysses Press, California.

Mehl-Madora, L. 2004, "Integrative approach to psychiatry," in *Integrative Medicine: Principles for Practice*, B. Kligler & R. Lee, eds., McGraw-Hill Medical, New York.

Meldolesi, J. & Pozzan, T. 1987, "Pathways of Ca2+ influx at the plasma membrane: voltage-, receptor-, and second messenger-operated channels," *Exp Cell Res*, vol. 171, no. 2, pp. 271-283.

Mentgen, J. L. 2001, "Healing touch," *Nurs Clin North Am*, vol. 36, no. 1, pp. 143-158.

Merritt, P. & Randall, D. 2002, *The Effect of Healing Touch and Other Forms of Energy Work on Cancer Pain. Healing Touch International Research Survey*, Healing Touch International, Lakewood, CO.

Micozzi, M. S. 2001, *Fundamentals of Complementary and Alternative Medicine*, 2 edn, Churchill Livingstone, Philadelphia.

Micozzi, M. S. & Singh, D. 2006, "Yoga," in *Fundamentals of complementary and Alternative Medicine*, M. S. Micozzi, ed., Sunders, Philadelphia.

Mikulecky, M., Moravcikova, C. & Czanner, S. 1996, "Lunisolar tidal waves, geomagnetic activity and epilepsy in the light of multivariate coherence," *Braz. J Med Biol Res*, vol. 29, no. 8, pp. 1069-1072.

Miller, A. 1998, "Dowsing: A review," *Network*, vol. 66, pp. 3-8.

Miller, M. W. 1986, "Extremely low frequency (ELF) electric fields: Experimental work on biological effects," in *CRC Handbook of Biological Effects of Electromagnetic Fields*, C. Polk & E. Postow, eds., CRC Press, Boca Raton, FL.

Mishler, E. G. 1981, "Viewpoint: Critical perspectives on the biomedical model," in *Social Contexts of Health, Illness, and Patients' care*, E. G. Mishler et al., eds., Cambridge University Press, Cambridge.

Mishler, E. G. 1984, *The Discourse of Medicine: Dialectics of Medical Interviews*, Ablex Publishing, Norwood, MA.

Mitchell, P. 1976, "Vectorial chemistry and the molecular mechanics of chemiosmotic coupling: Power transmission by proticity," *Biochem Soc Trans*, vol. 4, no. 3, pp. 399-430.

Mollon, P. Psychotherapists heal thing attitude. Paper presented to symposium on the Crucial factor in psychotherapy and psychoanalysis. Department of psychotherapy, Manchester Royal Infirmary, 4 November. 1991.

Montgomery, C. L. 1996, "The care-giving relationship: Paradoxical and transcendent aspects," *Altern Ther Health Med*, vol. 2, no. 2, pp. 52-57.

Morris, J. & Morris, W. 1998, *Reiki Hands That Heal* Red Wheel/Weiser, Massachusetts.

Murchie, G. 1979, *The Seven Mysteries of Life: Exploration in Science and Philosophy*, Houghton Mifflin, Boston.

Murphy, M., Donovan, S., & Taylor, E. 1997, *The Physical and Psychological Effects of Meditation: A Review of Contemporary Research with a Comprehensive Bibliography*, Institute of Noetic Sciences, Sausalito, CA.

Murugesan, R., Govindarajulu, N. & Bera, T. K. 2000, "Effect of selected yogic practices on the management of hypertension," *Indian J Physiol Pharmacol*, vol. 44, no. 2, pp. 207-210.

Myss, C. 1997, *Anatomy of the Spirit: The Seven Stages of Power and Healing*, Three Rivers Press, New York.

Naeser, M. A., Alexander, M. P., Stiassny-Eder, D., Galler, V., Hobbs, J., & Bachman, D. 1992, "Real versus sham acupuncture in the treatment of paralysis in acute stroke patients: A CT scan lesion site study," *J Neuro Rebabil*, vol. 6, no. 4, pp. 163-174.

National Center for Complementary and Alternative Medicine. Energy Medicine: An Overview [cited Oct 24, 2009]. Available from URL: http://nccam.nih.gov/health/whatiscam/energy/energymed.htm.

NCCAM. Energy Medicine: An Overview. NCCAM Publication No. D235 [cited Sep 10, 2009]. Available from URL: http://nccam.nih.gov/health/whatiscam/energy/energymed. htm.

Nelson, R. D. 1999, *The Physical Basis of International Healing Systems, Technical Report PEAR 99001*, Princeton Engineering Anomalies Research, Princeton University, Princeton.

Nespor, K. 1991, "Pain management and yoga," *Int J Psychosom*, vol. 38, no. 1-4, pp. 76-81.

Nield-Anderson, L. & Ameling, A. 2000, "The empowering nature of Reiki as a complementary therapy," *Holist Nurs Pract*, vol. 14, no. 3, pp. 21-29.

Nielson, A. & Hammerschlag, R. 2004, "Acupuncture and East Asian Medicine," in *Integrative Medicine: Principles for Practice*, B. Kligler & R. Lee, eds., McGrow Hill, New York.

Noontil, A. 1994, *The Body is the Barometer of the Soul: So Be Your Own Doctor II*, Annette Noontil, Nunawading, Vic.

Nurse Healers-Professional Associates 1992, *Guidelines for Teaching Therapeutic Touch by the Krieger/Kunz method: Intermediate Level*, Nurse Healers-Professional Associates, Philadelphia.

O'Mathuna, D. P. 2000, "Evidence-based practice and reviews of therapeutic touch," *J Nurs Scholarsh*, vol. 32, no. 3, pp. 279-285.

Ogden, J. 2004, *Health Psychology: A Textbook*, 3 edn, McGraw-Hill, New York.

Ohnishi, S. T., Ohnishi, T., Nishino, K., Tsurusaki, Y., & Yamaguchi, M. 2005, "Growth inhibition of cultured human liver carcinoma cells by Ki-energy (life-energy): Scientific evidence for Ki-effects on cancer cells," *Evid Based Complement Alternat Med*, vol. 2, no. 3, pp. 387-393.

Olson, K. & Hanson, J. 1997, "Using Reiki to manage pain: A preliminary report," *Cancer Prev Control*, vol. 1, no. 2, pp. 108-113.

Olson, K., Hanson, J. & Michaud, M. 2003, "A phase II trial of Reiki for the management of pain in advanced cancer patients," *J Pain Symptom. Manage.*, vol. 26, no. 5, pp. 990-997.

Oschman, J. L. 1984, "Structure and properties of ground substances," *American Zoologist*, vol. 24, pp. 199-215.

Oschman, J. L. 1989, "How the body maintains its shape," *Rolf Lines*, vol. 17, no. 3, p. 27.

Oschman, J. L. 1993, "Sensing solitons in soft tissues," *Guild News*, vol. 2, pp. 22-25.

Oschman, J. L. 1998, "What is healing energy? Part 6: Conclusions: is energy medicine the medicine of the future," *Journal of Bodywork and Movement Therapies*, vol. 2, no. 1, pp. 46-60.

Oschman, J. L. 2000a, *Energy medicine: The scientific basis*, Churchill Livingston, New York.

Oschman, J. L. 2000b, "The Electromagnetic Environment: Implications for bodywork part1; Environmental energies," *Journal of Bodywork and Movement Therapies*, vol. 4, no. 1, pp. 56-67.

Oschman, J. L. 2002, "Science and the Human Energy Field," *Reiki News*. Winter.

Oschman, J. L. & Oschman, N. H. 1994, *Physiological and Emotional Effects of Acupuncture Needle Insertion*, Proceedings of the Second Symposium of the Society for Acupuncture Research, Washington DC.

Oshman, J. L. 2007, "Energy medicine: the new paradigm," in *Complementary Therapies for Physical Therapy: A Clinical Decision-Making Approach*, J. E. Deutsch & E. Z. Anderson, eds.

Osterman, P. & Schwartz-Barcott, D. 1996, "Presence: four ways of being there," *Nurs Forum*, vol. 31, no. 2, pp. 23-30.

Ostrander, Sh. & Schroeder, L. 1984, *Psychic Discoveries Behind the Iron Curtain*, Prentice Hall Trade, Englewood Cliffs, NJ.

Pavesi, L. & Fauchet, P. M. 2008, *Biophotonics*, Springer, New York.

Peat, D. 1987, *Synchronicity: The Bridge Between Matter and Mind*, Bantam, Toronto.

Pengelley, E. T. & Asmundsen, S. J. 1971, "Annual biological clocks," *Scientific American*, vol. 224, p. 72.

Perry, F. S., Reichmanis, M., Marino, A. A., & Becker, R. O. 1981, "Environmental power-frequency magnetic fields and suicide," *Health Phys*, vol. 41, no. 2, pp. 267-277.

Persinger, M. A. 1996, "Enhancement of limbic seizures by nocturnal application of experimental magnetic fields that simulate the magnitude and morphology of increases in geomagnetic activity," *Int J Neurosci*, vol. 86, no. 3-4, pp. 271-280.

Peterson, I. 1997, "Getting physical with DNA. Stretching, twisting, prodding, and packing molecular strands," *Science News*, vol. 151, pp. 256-257.

Pienta, K. J. & Coffey, D. S. 1991, "Cellular harmonic information transfer through a tissue tensegrity-matrix system," *Med Hypotheses*, vol. 34, no. 1, pp. 88-95.

Post-White, J., Kinney, M. E., Savik, K., Gau, J. B., Wilcox, C. & Lerner, I. 2003, "Therapeutic massage and healing touch improve symptoms in cancer," *Integr Cancer Ther*, vol. 2, no. 4, pp. 332-344.

Potter, P. J. 2007, "Breast biopsy and distress: Feasibility of testing a Reiki intervention," *J Holist Nurs*, vol. 25, no. 4, pp. 238-248.

Preparata, G. 1995, *QED Coherence in Matter*, World Scientific Publishing, Singapore.

Quinn, J. F. 1984, "Therapeutic touch as energy exchange: Testing the theory," *ANS Adv Nurs Sci*, vol. 6, no. 2, pp. 42-49.

Quitkin, F. M., McGrath, P. J., Rabkin, J. G., Stewart, J. W., Harrison, W., Ross, D. C., Tricamo, E., Fleiss, J., Markowitz, J., & Klein, D. F. 1991, "Different types of placebo response in patients receiving antidepressants," *Am J Psychiatry*, vol. 148, no. 2, pp. 197-203.

Rajarshimuni, S. 1999, *Yoga: The Ultimate Attainment*, Jaico Publishing House, India.

Randler, Ch. 2009, "Morningness-Eveningness and Satisfaction with Life," *Social Indicators Research*, vol. 86, no. 2, pp. 297-302.

Rattemeyer, M., Popp, F. A., & Nagl, W. 1981, "Evidence of photon emission from DNA in living systems," *Naturwissenschaften*, vol. 68, no. 11, pp. 572-573.

Ray, U. S., Mukhopadhyaya, S., Purkayastha, S. S., Asnani, V., Tomer, O. S., Prashad, R., Thakur, L., & Selvamurthy, W. 2001, "Effect of yogic exercises on physical and mental health of young fellowship course trainees," *Indian J Physiol Pharmacol*, vol. 45, no. 1, pp. 37-53.

Reich, W. 1974, *The Function of the Orgasm; Sex-economic Problems of Biological Energy*, Touchstone, New York.

Rein, G. & McCarty, R. Modulation of DNA by coherent heart frequencies. Proceedings of the 3rd annual conference of the international society for the study of subtle Energies and Energy Medicine, Monterey, CA, June, 1993. 1993.

Riley, M. 2002, "Homeopathy," in *Complementary and Alternative Medicine Secrets*, W. Kohatsu, ed., Hanley & Belfus, Philadelphia.

Roberts, L., Ahmed, I., Hall, S. & Davison, A. 2009, "Intercessory prayer for the alleviation of ill health," *Cochrane Database Syst. Rev* no. 2, p. CD000368.

Roberts, R. & Groome, D. 2001, *Parapsychology: The Science of Unusual Experience*, Hodder Arnold, New York.

Rodgers, D. 2001, "Mind-Body Interventions," in *Fundamentals of Complementary and Alternative Medicine*, M. S. Micozzi, ed., Churchill Livingston, New York.

Roethlisberger, F. J. & Dickson, W. J. 1939, *Management and the Worker: An Account of a Research Program Conducted by Western Electric Company*, Harvard University Press, Cambridge.

Rogers, C. R., Kirschenbaum, H., & Henderson, V. L. 1990, *The Carl Rogers Reader*, Constable, London.

Rogers, M. E. 1970, *An Introduction to the Theoretical Basis of Nursing*, Davis, Philadelphia.

Rogers, M. E. 1983, *The Science of Unitary Human Being: A Paradigm for Nursing*, Davis, Philadelphia.

Rogers, M. E. 1989, "Science of unitary human beings: A paradigm for nursing," in *Family health: A Theoretical Approach to Nursing Care*, I. W. Clements & F. B. Roberts, eds., Wiley, New York.

Rohrlich, F. 1983, "Facing Quantum Mechanical Reality," *Science*, vol. 221, no. 4617, pp. 1251-1255.

Rolf, I. P. 1962, "Structural integration. Gravity: an unexplored factor in a more human use of human beings," *Philosophy and the Sciences*, vol. 1, pp. 3-20.

Ronan, C. A. 1983, *The Cambridge Illustrated History of the World's Science*, Cambridge University Press, Cambridge.

Rood, Y. R., Bogaards, M., Goulmy, E., & Houwelingen, H. C. 1993, "The effects of stress and relaxation on the in vitro immune response in man: a meta-analytic study," *J Behav Med*, vol. 16, no. 2, pp. 163-181.

Rosenthal, R. 1994, "Interpersonal expectancy effects: A thirty-year perspective," *Current Directions in Psychological Science*, vol. 3, pp. 176-179.

Rotan, L. W. & Ospina-Kammerer, V. 2007, *MindBody Medicine. Foundations and Practical Applications*, Routledge, New York.

Rowan, J. 2005, *The Transpersonal: Spirituality in Psychotherapy and Counselling*, Rutledge, New York.

Rubik, B., Becker, R. O., Flower, R. G., Hazlewood, C. F., Liboff, A. R., & Walleczek, J. 1994, "Bioelectromagnetics applications in medicine. NIH Publication No. 94-066," in *Alternative Medicine-Expanding Medical Horizons*, Government Printing Office, Washington DC.

Rubik, B., Brooks, A. J., & Schwartz, G. E. 2006, "In vitro effect of Reiki treatment on bacterial cultures: Role of experimental context and practitioner well-being," *J Altern Complement Med*, vol. 12, no. 1, pp. 7-13.

Ruhl, T. S. 2002, "Spiritual informed consent for CAM," *Arch Intern Med*, vol. 162, no. 8, pp. 943-944.

Russell, H. 2002, "Yoga," in *Complementary and Alternative Medicine Secrets*, W. Kohatsu, ed., Hanley & Belfus, Philadelphia.

Sancier, K. M. 1996, "Medical applications of Qigong," *Altern. Ther Health Med*, vol. 2, no. 1, pp. 40-46.

Sarafino, E. P. Health Psychology: Biopsychosocial Interactions. 2005. Wiley.

Schlitz, M. 2004, "Intentional Healing: Exploring the Extended Reaches of Consciousness," *Subtle Energies & Energy Medicine*, vol. 14, no. 1, pp. 1-18.

Schlitz, M. & Braud, W. 1985, "Reiki-Plus natural healing: an ethnographic/experimental study," *PSI Research*, vol. 4, no. 3, pp. 100-123.

Schlitz, M. & Braud, W. 1997, "Distant intentionality and healing: assessing the evidence," *Altern Ther Health Med*, vol. 3, no. 6, pp. 62-73.

Schlitz, M. & Haight, J. M. 1984, "Remote viewing revisited: An intrasubject replication," *Journal of Parapsychology*, vol. 48, pp. 39-49.

Schrödinger, E. 1967, "What is life? The physical aspect of the living cell and mind and matter," Cambridge University Press, Cambridge.

Schuman, W. O. & Knig, H. 1954, "-ber die Beobachtung von Atmospheics bei geringstein Frequenzen," *Naturwissenschaften*, vol. 41, p. 183.

Schwartz, S., De Mattei, R., Brame, E., & Spottiswoode, J. 1991, "Infrared spectra alteration in water proximate to the palms of therapeutic practitioners," *Subtle Energies*, vol. 1, pp. 43-54.

Selye, H. 1978, *The Stress of Life* McGraw-Hill, New York.

Sentman, D. D. 1995, "Schumann resonances," in *Handbook of Atmospheric Electrodynamics*, H. Volland, ed., CRC Press, Boca Raton.

Seto, A., Kusaka, C., Nakazato, S., Huang, W. R., Sato, T., Hisamitsu, T. & Takeshige, C. 1992, "Detection of extraordinary large bio-magnetic field strength from human hand during external Qi emission," *Acupunct Electrother Res*, vol. 17, no. 2, pp. 75-94.

Shah, S., Ogden, A. T., Pettker, C. M., Raffo, A., Itescu, S., & Oz, M. C. 1999, "A study of the effect of energy healing on in vitro tumor cell proliferation," *J Altern Complement Med*, vol. 5, no. 4, pp. 359-365.

Shamlou, S. 2002, *Clinical Psychology*, Roshd, Tehran.

Shapira, M. Y., Berkman, N., Ben-David, G., Avital, A., Bardach, E., & Breuer, R. 2002, "Short-term acupuncture therapy is of no benefit in patients with moderate persistent asthma," *Chest*, vol. 121, no. 5, pp. 1396-1400.

Shapiro, A. K. & Shapiro, E. 1997, *The Powerful Placebo: From Ancient Priest to Modern Physician*, The Johns Hopkins University Press, Baltimore, MD.

Sharifi, M. 2003, "The role of acupuncture in health delivery system: II-mechanisms," *Iraninan Journal of Higher Health (Salamat-e-Bartar)*, vol. 2, no. 3, pp. 119-137.

Shen, X. & Van Wijk, R. 2006, *Biophotonics: Optical Science and Engineering for the 21st Century* Springer, New York.

Sherman, K. J., Cherkin, D. C., Erro, J., Miglioretti, D. L., & Deyo, R. A. 2005, "Comparing yoga, exercise, and a self-care book for chronic low back pain: a randomized, controlled trial," *Ann Intern Med*, vol. 143, no. 12, pp. 849-856.

Shiflett, S. C., Nayak, S., Bid, C., Miles, P., & Agostinelli, S. 2002, "Effect of Reiki treatments on functional recovery in patients in poststroke rehabilitation: A pilot study," *J Altern Complement Med*, vol. 8, no. 6, pp. 755-763.

Shore, A. G. 2004, "Long-term effects of energetic healing on symptoms of psychological depression and self-perceived stress," *Altern Ther Health Med*, vol. 10, no.3, pp. 42-48.

Sierpina, V. S. & Sierpina, M. 2004, "Spirituality and health," in *Integrative medicine; Principles for Practices*, B. Kligler & R. Lee, eds., McGraw-Hill, New York.

Simson, S. P. & Straus, M. C. 1998, *Horticulture as Therapy: Principles and Practice*, The Haworth Press, Binghamton.

Sisken, B. F. & Walker, J. 1995, "Therapeutic aspects of electromagnetic fields for soft-tissue healing," in *Electromagnetic fields*, M. Blank, ed., American Chemical Society, Washington DC.

Skilnand, E., Fossen, D., & Heiberg, E. 2002, "Acupuncture in the management of pain in labor," *Acta Obstet Gynecol Scand*, vol. 81, no. 10, pp. 943-948.

Slater, V. E. 2000, "Energetic healing," in *Holistic Nursing: A Handbook for Practice*, 3 edn, B. M. Dossey & L. Keegan, eds., Aspen Publishers, Gaithersburg, MD.

Smith, C. W. 1987, "Electromagnetic effects in humans," in *Biological Coherence and Response to External Stimuli*, H. Frhlich, ed., Springer, Berlin.

Smith, C. W. 1994, "Biological effects of weak electromagnetic fields," in *Bioelectrodynamics and Biocommunication*, H. Mae-Wan, F. A. Popp, & U. Warnke, eds., World Scientific Publishing Company, Singapore.

Smith, C. W. & Best, S. 1989, *Electromagnetic Man: Health and Hazard in the Electrical Environment*, Palgrave Macmillan, London.

Smith, D. W. & Broida, J. P. 2007, "Pandimensional field pattern changes in healers and healees: Experiencing therapeutic touch," *J Holist Nurs*, vol. 25, no. 4, pp. 217-225.

So, D. W. 2002, "Acupuncture outcomes, expectations, patient—provider relationship, and the placebo effect: Implications for health promotion," *Am J Public Health*, vol. 92, no. 10, pp. 1662-1667.

Sperry, R. W. 1969, "A modified concept of consciousness," *Psychol Rev*, vol. 76, no. 6, pp. 532-536.

Sprangers, M. A., Van Dam, F. S., Broersen, J., Lodder, L., Wever, L., Visser, M. R., Oosterveld, P., & Smets, E. M. 1999, "Revealing response shift in longitudinal research on fatigue—the use of the thentest approach," *Acta Oncol*, vol. 38, no. 6, pp. 709-718.

Staunton, T. 2002, *Body psychotherapy*, Brunner-Routledge, New York.

Stein, D. 2000, *Essential Reiki, A Complete Guide to an Ancient Healing Art*, Crossing Press, New York.

Stoupel, E., Goldenfeld, M., Shimshoni, M., & Siegel, R. 1993, "Intraocular pressure (IOP) in relation to four levels of daily geomagnetic and extreme yearly solar activity," *Int J Biometeorol*, vol. 37, no. 1, pp. 42-45.

Stoupel, E., Martfel, J. N., & Rotenberg, Z. 1994, "Paroxysmal atrial fibrillation and stroke (cerebrovascular accidents) in males and females above and below age 65 on days of different geomagnetic activity levels," *J Basic Clin Physiol Pharmacol*, vol. 5, no. 3-4, pp. 315-329.

Stoupel, E., Wittenberg, C., Zabludowski, J., & Boner, G. 1995, "Ambulatory blood pressure monitoring in patients with hypertension on days of high and low geomagnetic activity," *J Hum Hypertens*, vol. 9, no. 4, pp. 293-294.

Straus, J. L. & von Ammon, C. S. 1996, "Placebo effects. Issues for clinical practice in psychiatry and medicine," *Psychosomatics*, vol. 37, no.4, pp. 315-326.

Suarez, M., Raffaelli, M. & O'Leary, A. 1996, "Use of folk healing practices by HIV-infected Hispanics living in the United States," *AIDS Care*, vol. 8, no. 6, pp. 683-690.

Sun, Q. & Zhao, L. Clinical Observation of Qigang as a therapeutic aid for advanced. Proceedings, Second World Conf on *Academic Exchange of Medical Qigong*, Beijing, China. 1993.

Szent-Gyorgyi, A. 1941, "Toward a new biochemistry?" *Science*, vol. 93, no. 2426, pp. 609-611.

Szent-Gyrgyi, A. 1988, "To see what everyone has seen, to think what no one has thought," *Biological Bulletin*, vol. 175, pp. 191-240.

Takahashi, K., Kaneko, I., Date, M., & Fukada, E. 1986, "Effect of pulsing electromagnetic fields on DNA synthesis in mammalian cells in culture," *Experientia*, vol. 42, no. 2, pp. 185-186.

Tang, T., Kiang, J. G., & Cox, B. M. 1994, "Opioids acting through delta receptors elicit a transient increase in the intracellular free calcium concentration in dorsal root ganglion—neuroblastoma hybrid ND8-47 cells," *J Pharmacol Exp Ther*, vol. 270, no. 1, pp. 40-46.

Targ, E. 2002, "Research methodology for studies of prayer and distant healing," *Complement Ther Nurs Midwifery*, vol. 8, no. 1, pp. 29-41.

Thoms, L. 2003, "Back to our roots for serenity?" *Psychologist*, vol. 17, no. 7, pp. 356-357.

Tiller, W. A. 2002, "The Real World of Modern Science, Medicine, and Qigong," *Bulletin of Science, Technology and Society*, vol. 22, no. 5, pp. 352-361.

Tloczynski, J. & Fritzsch, S. 2002, "Intercessory prayer in psychological well-being: using a multiple-baseline, across-subjects design," *Psychol Rep*, vol. 91, no. 3 Pt 1, pp. 731-741.

Todaro-Franceschi, V. 1999, *The enigma of energy: where science and religion converge*, Cross-Road Publishing, New York.

Tornatore, N. V. & Tornatore, R. 1977, "The paranormal event in psychotherapy," *Psychic*, vol. July, pp. 34-37.

Trapp, M. J. & Bulbrook, M. J. 1996a, *Healing Touch level I notebook*, North Carolina Center for Healing Touch, Carrboro.

Trapp, M. J. & Bulbrook, M. J. 1996b, *Healing Touch level II notebook*, North Carolina Center for Healing Touch, Carrboro.

Tromp, S. 1968, "Review of the possible physiological causes of dowsing," *International Journal of Parapsychology*, vol. 10, no. 4, pp. 363-391.

Tse, S. K. & Bailey, D. M. 1992, "Tai chi and postural control in the well elderly," *Am J Occup Ther*, vol. 46, no. 4, pp. 295-300.

Uexkull, T.V. & Pauli H.G. 1986, *The Mind-Body Problem in Medicine,* Advances, Advancement of Health, vol. 8, no.4, pp. 158-174

Udupa, K. N. 1983, "Yoga and meditation for mental health," in *Traditional Medicine and Health-Care Coverage. A Reader for Health Administrators and Practitioners*, R. H. Bannerman, J. Burton & Ch. Wen-Chieh, eds., World Health Organization, Geneva.

Ulrich, R. S. 1984, "View through a window may influence recovery from surgery," *Science*, vol. 224, no. 4647, pp. 420-421.

Usenko, G. A. & Panin, L. E. 1993, "[Blood system reactions in flight operators with high and low levels of anxiousness during geomagnetic disturbances]," *Aviakosm Ekolog Med*, vol. 27, no. 2, pp. 39-44.

Van Sell, S. L. 1996, "Reiki: An ancient touch therapy," *RN*, vol. 59, no. 2, pp. 57-59.

Vaughan, F. E. 1986, *The Inward Arc: Healing and Wholeness in Psychotherapy and Spirituality*, Shambhala Publications, California.

Vincent, C. & Furnham, A.1996, "Why do patients turn to complementary medicine? An empirical study," *Br J Clin Psychol*, vol. 35 (Pt 1), pp. 37-48.

Vitale, A. 2007, "An integrative review of Reiki touch therapy research," *Holist Nurs Pract*, vol. 21, no. 4, pp. 167-179.

Vitale, A. T. & O'Connor, P. C. 2006, "The effect of Reiki on pain and anxiety in women with abdominal hysterectomies: a quasi-experimental pilot study," *Holist Nurs Pract*, vol. 20, no. 6, pp. 263-272.

Volland, H. 1984, *Handbook of Atmospheric Electrodynamics*, CRC Press, Boca Raton.

Volland, H. 1995, *Handbook of Atmospheric Electrodynamics*, CRC Press, Bonn.

Von Aschoff, D. Geopathische zonenphysikalische Grundlage der Krebsentstehung. Presented at the International Congress ZDN, Essen, 19 October 1985. Mehr Wisen Buch-Deinst, Dusseldorf. 1985.

Wachtel, H. 1995, "Comparison of Endogenous Currents in and Around Cells with Those Induced by Exogenous Extremely Low Frequency Magnetic Fields," *Advances in Chemistry*, vol. 250, pp. 99-107.

Walach, H. 2001, "The efficacy paradox in randomized controlled trials of CAM and elsewhere: beware of the placebo trap," *J Altern Complement Med*, vol. 7, no. 3, pp. 213-218.

Walach, H., Schmidt, S., Dirhold, T., & Nosch, S. 2002, "The effects of a caffeine placebo and suggestion on blood pressure, heart rate, well-being and cognitive performance," *Int J Psychophysiol*, vol. 43, no. 3, pp. 247-260.

Wallenstein, G. V. 1994, "A model of the electrophysiological properties of nucleus reticularis thalami neurons," *Biophys J*, vol. 66, no. 4, pp. 978-988.

Wang, C., Xu, D., Qian, Y., & Shi, W., 1993. Effects of Qigang on preventing stroke and alleviating the multiple cerebro-cardiovascular risk factors: a follow-up report on 242 hypertensive case over 30 years. Proceedings from the second world conference for Academic Exchange of Medical Qigang. Bijing:123-124.

Ward, R. R. 1972, *The Living Clocks* Signet, New York.

Wardell, D. W. 2000, "Trauma Release Technique as Taught and Experienced in the Healing Touch Program," *Alternative and Complementary Therapies*, vol. 6, no. 1, pp. 20-27.

Wardell, D. W. 2001, "Spiritually of Healing Touch Participants," *Journal of Holistic Nursing*, vol. 19, pp. 71-86.

Wardell, D. W. & Engebretson, J. 2001, "Ethical principles applied to complementary healing," *J Holist Nurs*, vol. 19, no. 4, pp. 318-334.

Wardell, D. W. & Engebretson, J. C. 2006, "Taxonomy of Spiritual Experience," *Journal of Religion and Health*, vol. 45, no. 2, pp. 215-233.

Wardell, D. W. & Weymouth, K. F. 2004, "Review of studies of healing touch," *J Nurs. Scholarsh.*, vol. 36, no. 2, pp. 147-154.

Watson, L. 1999, *Supernature* Coronet Books, London.

Weeks, J. 2001, in *Integrating Complementary Medicine into Health Systems*, N. Faass, ed., Aspen Publishers, Philadelphia.

West, W. 1997, "Integrating counselling, psychotherapy and healing: An inquiry into counsellors and psychotherapists whose work includes healing," *British Journal of Guidance & Counselling*, vol. 25, no. 3, pp. 291-311.

West, W. 2000, *Psychotherapy & Spirituality: Crossing the Line between Therapy and Religion* Sage Publications, London.

Wetzel, W. S. 1993, "Healing touch as a nursing intervention: wound infection following cesarean birth—an anecdotal case study," *J Holist Nurs*, vol. 11, no. 3, pp. 277-285.

Weymouth, K. & Sandberg-Lewis, S. 2000, "Comparing the efficacy of healing touch and chiropractic adjustment in treating chronic low back pain: A pilot study," *Healing Touch Newsletter*, vol. 00, no. 3, pp. 7-8.

Wheeler-Robins, J. 1999, *Psychoneuroimmunology and healing touch in HIV disease. Unpublished doctoral dissertation* Virginia Commonwealth University, Richmond, VA.

Whelan, K. M. & Wishnia, G. S. 2003, "Reiki therapy: the benefits to a nurse/Reiki practitioner," *Holist. Nurs. Pract.*, vol. 17, no. 4, pp. 209-217.

WHO 2001, *Legal Status of Traditional Medicine and Complementary/Alternative Medicine: A Worldwide Review* World Health Organization, Geneva.

Wilber, K. 1977, *The Spectrum of Consciousness* Theosophical Publishing Hoase, New York.

Wilber, K. 1990, "Two Patterns of Transcendence: A Reply to Washburn," *Journal of Humanistic Psychology*, vol. 30, no. 3, pp. 113-136.

Wilkinson, D. 2002, *The clinical effectiveness of healing touch on HIV-infected individuals* Tennessee State University, Nashville, TN.

Williams, K. A., Petronis, J., Smith, D., Goodrich, D., Wu, J., Ravi, N., Doyle, E. J. Jr., Gregory, J. R., Munoz, K. M., Gross, R., & Steinberg, L. 2005, "Effect of Iyengar yoga therapy for chronic low back pain," *Pain*, vol. 115, no. 1-2, pp. 107-117.

Winstead-Fry, P. & Kijek, J. 1999, "An integrative review and meta-analysis of therapeutic touch research," *Altern Ther Health Med*, vol. 5, no. 6, pp. 58-67.

Wirth, D. P., Barrett, M. J. & Eidelman, W. S. 1994, "Non-contact therapeutic touch and wound re-epithelialization: an extension of previous research," *Compl Ther Med*, vol. 2, pp. 187-192.

Wirth, D. P., Brennan, D. R., Levine, R. J. & Rodriguez, C. M. 1993, "The effect of complementary healing therapy on postoperative pain after surgical removal of impacted third molar teeth," *Complement Ther Med*, vol. 1, pp. 133-138.

Wirth, D. P., Richardson, J. T., & Eidelman, W. S. 1996, "Wound healing and complementary therapies: a review," *J Altern Complement Med*, vol. 2, no. 4, pp. 493-502.

Wiseman, R. & Schlitz, M. 1997, "Experimenter effects and the remote detection of staring," *Journal of Parapsychology*, vol. 61, pp. 197-208.

Wiseman, N. & Ellis, A. 1985, *Fundamentals of Chinese Medicine*, Paradigm Publication, Brookline.

Wisneski, L. A. 1997, "A unified energy field theory of physiology and healing," *Stress Med*, vol. 13, pp. 259-265.

Wlkinson, D. 2002, *The Clinical Effectiveness of Healing Touch on HIV-Infected Individuals*, Tennessee State University, Nashville, TN.

Wolsko, P. M., Eisenberg, D. M., Davis, R. B., & Phillips, R. S. 2004, "Use of mind-body medical therapies," *J Gen Intern Med*, vol. 19, no. 1, pp. 43-50.

Wu, C. 1997, "A magnet for a future atom smasher," *Science News*, vol. 151, no. 31May, p. 340.

Xu, D. & Wang, C. Clinical study of delaying effect on senility of hypertensive patients by practicing "Yang Jing Yi Gong." Proceedings from the fifth international symposium on Qigang, Shanghai; 1994.

Yan, X., Shen, H., Zaharia, M., Wang, J., Wolf, D., Li, F., Lee, G. D., & Cao, W. 2004, "Involvement of phosphatidylinositol 3-kinase and insulin-like growth factor-I in YXLST-mediated neuroprotection," *Brain Res*, vol. 1006, no. 2, pp. 198-206.

Yang, K. H., Kim, Y. H. & Lee, M. S. 2005, "Efficacy of Qi therapy (external Qigong) for elderly people with chronic pain," *Int J Neurosci*, vol. 115, no. 7, pp. 949-963.

Zachariae, R., Hojgaard, L., Zachariae, C., Vaeth, M., Bang, B., & Skov, L. 2005, "The effect of spiritual healing on in vitro tumour cell proliferation and viability—an experimental study," *Br J Cancer*, vol. 93, no. 5, pp. 538-543.

Zachariae, R., Kristensen, J. S., Hokland, P., Ellegaard, J., Metze, E., & Hokland, M. 1990, "Effect of psychological intervention in the form of relaxation and guided imagery on cellular immune function in normal healthy subjects. An overview," *Psychother Psychosom*, vol. 54, no. 1, pp. 32-39.

Zamarra, J. W., Schneider, R. H., Besseghini, I., Robinson, D. K., & Salerno, J. W. 1996, "Usefulness of the transcendental meditation program in the treatment of patients with coronary artery disease," *Am J Cardiol*, vol. 77, no. 10, pp. 867-870.

Zhang, Y. Y. 1993, *Zhang Guo Qigong Da Quan* Tien Tsin Ren Min Publishing Co., Tien Tsin.

Zimmerman, J. 1990, "Laying-on-of-hands healing and therapeutic touch: a testable theory," *BEMI Currents, Journal of the Bio-Electro-Magnetics Institute*, vol. 2, no. 1, pp. 8-17.

Zimmerman, J. E. & Harding, J. T. 1970, "Design and operation of stable rf-biased superconducting point-contact quantum devices, and a note on the properties of perfectly clean metal contacts," *Journal of Applied Physics*, vol. 41, pp. 1572-1580.

Index

C